The Emetophobia Survival Guide

of related interest

Conquer Your Emetophobia
Advice from a Therapist Who Overcame the Fear of Vomiting
Anna S. Christie
ISBN 978 1 80501 776 9
eISBN 978 1 80501 777 6

Free Yourself from Emetophobia
A CBT Self-Help Guide for a Fear of Vomiting
Alexandra Keyes and David Veale
ISBN 978 1 78775 331 0
eISBN 978 1 78775 332 7

Bodie and the Ghost Showdown
An Emetophobia Story
Dr Ffion Jones
Illustrated by Kara McHale
ISBN 978 1 80501 985 5
eISBN 978 1 80501 986 2

Facing Mighty Fears about Throwing Up
Dawn Huebner, PhD
Illustrated by Liza Stevens
ISBN 978 1 78775 925 1
eISBN 978 1 78775 926 8
Dr. Dawn's Mini Books about Mighty Fears collection

The Emetophobia Survival Guide

A Young Person's Handbook for Recovery

EMMA INNES

Foreword by Anna S. Christie

Jessica Kingsley Publishers
London and Philadelphia

First published in Great Britain in 2027 by Jessica Kingsley Publishers
An imprint of John Murray Publishing Group

1

Front cover image source: Shutterstock®.

A CIP catalogue record for this title is available from the British Library and the Library of Congress

ISBN 978 1 39983 146 8
eISBN 978 1 39983 147 5

Printed and bound in Great Britain by Clays Ltd

Jessica Kingsley Publishers' policy is to use papers that are natural, renewable and recyclable products and made from wood grown in sustainable forests. The logging and manufacturing processes are expected to conform to the environmental regulations of the country of origin.

Jessica Kingsley Publishers
Carmelite House
50 Victoria Embankment
London EC4Y 0DZ

www.jkp.com

John Murray Publishing Group
Part of Hodder & Stoughton Ltd
An Hachette Company

The authorised representative in the EEA is Hachette Ireland,
8 Castlecourt Centre, Dublin 15, D15 XTP3, Ireland (email: info@hbgi.ie)

Contents

Foreword

Anna S. Christie, licensed psychotherapist and emetophobia specialist

Emetophobia is one of the least understood yet most life-altering anxiety disorders I have ever encountered in clinical practice. Despite its prevalence, it remains largely unspoken about – hidden beneath layers of shame, secrecy and profound misunderstanding. For many young people, the fear of vomiting becomes a battle they navigate alone without accurate information, guidance or support. This is precisely why *The Emetophobia Survival Guide* is such an important book.

The most difficult years to live with emetophobia can be the teenage and college-age stages. Emma Innes has been there and understands. She has created a resource that is not only accessible and relatable but also accurate and insightful. Her writing reflects a deep understanding of the things that drive emetophobia: constant worry over bodily cues, the fear of uncertainty, the overestimation of threat, the reliance on safety behaviours and the profound avoidance that narrows a young person's world.

Emma's personal experience gives her a unique vantage point. She captures the emotional landscape of emetophobia with nuance: the constant anticipatory anxiety, the exhaustion of continuous monitoring, the difficulties with food, the challenges in school and social environments and the pervasive belief that something terrible could happen at any moment. She gives language to the internal turmoil that so many young people cannot yet describe.

One of the most significant strengths of this book is that it reduces isolation. Many of my patients and social media followers have never met anyone else with this phobia, and they often believe they are 'the only one' who thinks or behaves this way. The stories, examples and explanations throughout this guide make it abundantly clear that they are not alone – and that their symptoms are both understandable and treatable.

Clinically, Emma's descriptions align with what the (meagre) amount of research into emetophobia has shown:

- Emetophobia almost always begins in childhood.
- It can sometimes begin after a period of heightened stress, illness or loss of perceived bodily control.
- It is maintained by safety behaviours, avoidance, reassurance-seeking and misinterpretation of harmless bodily sensations.
- It is not a sign of weakness, and it is nobody's fault.

Most importantly, emetophobia is responsive to evidence-based treatment. With appropriate therapeutic support – and cognitive behavioural therapy with gradual exposure and response prevention (ERP) – young people can overcome the fear that has been shaping their lives so that they can enter adulthood with as much hope and joy as everyone else.

Emma covers every aspect of living with emetophobia: food, friends, school, dating, travel, family, digital life, treatment, and the delicate art of taking care of yourself when everything feels overwhelming. Her guidance is practical, grounded, research-informed and – most importantly – shaped by lived experience. Young people will feel understood in these pages. Parents, teachers and therapists will finally have a resource they can hand to a struggling teen and say, 'This will help.'

For the young person holding this book, perhaps feeling anxious even beginning to read about a topic they work so hard to avoid, I want to say this clearly: you are safe, you are understood, and you are absolutely capable of getting better. Emetophobia can feel overwhelming, but it does not define you. With compassion, knowledge and the right tools – which you will find in these pages – you can build a life that is not governed by fear. Many before you have recovered, and you can too. Let this book be your companion as you begin that journey. With Emma's steady voice in your ear and the right support around you, recovery is not just possible – it is likely.

I am honoured to introduce *The Emetophobia Survival Guide* to you. May it be a source of clarity, courage and genuine hope on your path towards recovery.

Acknowledgements

Thank you to my editor, Jane Evans at Jessica Kingsley Publishers, for recognising the importance of raising awareness of emetophobia, and for giving me the opportunity to do my bit. Also, for making my first experience of traditional publishing so enjoyable. Thank you to Will Moran for all their kind and efficient help and support and to Carys Homer, Faye Collins, Kath Mackrill, Claire Shewbridge, Grażyna Martins, Ros Bird, Michaela O'Callaghan and the wider team at Jessica Kingsley.

Thank you to Anna Christie for taking the time to read the manuscript of this book and give her expert insights. Also, for generously writing the foreword to *The Emetophobia Survival Guide*.

Thank you to Dr Guy Benison-Horner for sharing his NHS GP wisdom with me, and to my lovely case studies Becky, Zoe, Zara, Ellie and Remy for allowing me to hear, and share, their stories.

Finally, thank you to the generous people who read the early drafts of *The Emetophobia Survival Guide* and helped me bash it into shape – Anthea Church, Florence George, James Innes and Caroline Phippen.

INTRODUCTION: EMMA AND EMETOPHOBIA

Emetophobia ruined my youth. I don't want it to do the same to yours.

Constant nausea, violent shaking and extreme anxiety. This was my experience of teenage life. Where there should have been parties, hanging out with friends and increasing independence, I had panic attacks, food avoidance and antidepressants.

The cause? Emetophobia. The extreme and debilitating phobia of vomiting.

My experience

I developed emetophobia when I was fourteen after a bout of illness in Mauritius. This experience flipped me from healthy-but-a-bit-highly-strung, to a full-blown, debilitating anxiety disorder. It left me feeling trapped. I felt like I could never be safe again because I couldn't escape my body, which was the thing I feared the most.

From age fourteen, the phobia got progressively worse throughout the rest of my time at school as exam pressure built and teenage hormones raged. By the time I was eighteen and in the final year of school, I was having extended panic attacks every morning, which sometimes caused retching, and always teeth-clatteringly-bad shaking. I felt sick constantly, could only eat a very small range of unhealthy, processed foods, avoided leaving home and was underweight and malnourished.

Dodging various threats of hospitalisation, I staggered through to the end of my exams. Suddenly I found myself free of school, but hopelessly unwell and with a year – my gap year – to fix myself if I wanted to take up the place I'd been offered at the University of Cambridge.

A year of sleeping, resting, visiting psychiatrists and taking ever higher doses of antidepressants followed. Miraculously, with the meds onboard, a bit of cognitive behavioural therapy (CBT) under my belt, and some serious rest and recuperation, I went on to have a wonderful time at university.

Thanks, I assume, to maturing a bit, being in a different environment, with different people, and a different lifestyle – not to mention a generous helping of selective serotonin reuptake inhibitors (SSRIs) – I got better and better while I was there. By the time I left three years later, I not only had a degree and a boyfriend (who is now my husband), but I was a healthy weight, was able to eat, party and travel, and was starting to think about coming off the medication.

So, that's the very brief potted history of my experience of emetophobia.

I'm now thirty-six and how's my relationship with emetophobia? Well, I'd like to claim I'm cured, but that wouldn't be true. I'm hugely better than I was, but I'm still working on the lingering anxieties and habits which are so heavily ingrained in me. That's okay, though, because it's no longer debilitating, and it no longer causes me frequent distress. Crucially, it also no longer has an impact on my physical health and wellbeing.

Through writing *The Emetophobia Survival Guide*, and sharing my experience and the things I've learned, I hope to be able to help you achieve a similar, if not better, improvement in your battle with this invisible but mighty foe.

I also hope to show you that you are not alone, you aren't crazy and while emetophobia causes huge suffering, there is light at the end of the tunnel.

The book

In this book, I'm going to explore what emetophobia is, how it's treated, and how it can impact people's relationships, health, wellbeing, education, careers and ability to eat. With reference to my own experience, I'll give tips and advice on how to navigate all these areas of life while living with the phobia. I will also cover how to stay safe in the digital world, how to look after yourself and, crucially, how to keep having FUN while living with this diagnosable and treatable condition.

All the information in *The Emetophobia Survival Guide* is based on a combination of my own experience of living with, and recovering from, emetophobia, suggestions from experts treating and researching the condition, and the thoughts of a few people who've kindly shared their experiences of having emetophobia in their teen years.

Everyone's experience of emetophobia, how they developed it and their journey to recovery is different but I hope you find this book informative and helpful.

Please forgive the fact I've written in my own, authentic voice in a bid to make it accessible and personable. I'm aware I have a dry sense of humour – it's my way of dealing with things – but please don't take this as me belittling emetophobia, or the suffering it causes, in any way.

Please also forgive the female slant to elements of the book – it covers my experience of living with emetophobia as a teenage girl, and, due to the difficulties in finding men with emetophobia who want to share their story, the case studies included are all women. This reflects the fact that ninety percent of people with emetophobia are female. However, males with emetophobia generally experience a very similar range of symptoms to females and, of course, the treatment is the same regardless of gender. So please plough on – the book is just as relevant to boys and young men as it is to girls and women.

You may find this a tricky book to read at times, especially if it's making you face up to, and engage with, the thing you fear most. This is completely understandable – you're being very brave just picking it up. Simply by reading about the condition, you're taking the first steps towards conquering it. If you find it difficult to read, you might consider tackling just one chapter a day, taking regular breaks from reading, or rewarding yourself in some way for getting through each section. A cup of tea and a biscuit, maybe?

You may also find it helpful to discuss what you've read with someone you trust. If so, you could consider offering the book to friends or relatives to help them understand what it's like to live with emetophobia, and to give them an idea of how they can best support you. They will be better placed to talk through the book with you if they've also read it.

Finally...

Emetophobia is an extremely difficult condition to live with. Experts Dr David Russ and Anna Christie say, 'Emetophobia is not just being grossed out by or not liking to vomit, it is wholly debilitating, ruining the lives of those who suffer from it.'[1]

It can cause great distress, and it isn't easy to overcome but with courage, perseverance and patience, emetophobia can be effectively treated and you can get your life back.

Even though I don't know you, I have been rooting for you while writing this book and I sincerely hope it will help you in your recovery – I would love to hear how you get on.

Emma Innes
September 2025

Chapter 1

WHAT EVEN IS THIS THING?

The definitions

Let's start with the basics. What actually is emetophobia? To be honest, most people – including many people who have it – have never heard of the condition and haven't got a clue what it is. We need to plug this knowledge gap before we do anything else, because the first step towards winning any battle is getting to know your enemy. So here goes...

The official definition: 'Emetophobia is a fear of vomiting or seeing others being sick. Those who experience emetophobia may also fear being out of control while they are being sick or fear being sick in public, which can trigger avoidance behaviours.'[1]

My definition: Emetophobia is a powerful internal dictator who cannot be reasoned with and will not bow down to basic common sense. Kind of like a toddler having a tantrum. But one that only exists inside your own head.

No, okay, let's be sensible. It's a fear of vomit so overwhelming that it outweighs absolutely everything else in life. It can trump friendships, romantic relationships, your education or career goals, your desire to show basic politeness at meals, your capacity to travel, and even your need to provide your body with vital nourishment.

It can control what you are able to eat, drink, do, wear and be. It causes devastating levels of near-constant anxiety and can detrimentally impact every element of a person's wellbeing and quality of life.

Sounds brutal, and it is. Trust me, I know.

Psychologists Dr Alexandra Keyes and Professor David Veale are world experts on emetophobia. They say, 'Emetophobia is likely to result in extreme anxiety and distress, avoidance of many day-to-day activities, and changes in behaviour and attention.'[2] They add that the phobia can have a devastating impact on a person's life.

The symptoms

So that's what it is. But what is it like to live with? What symptoms does it cause on a day-to-day basis? The list of possible signs and symptoms of this little-known, but relatively common, phobia – which is also known as specific fear of vomiting[3] – is very long. It differs from person to person, but it includes:

- anxiety
- performing 'safety-seeking behaviours'
- constant worry about vomiting and intrusive thoughts about being sick

- panic attacks
- disordered eating.

I could go on.

To be officially diagnosed with the phobia, you must have had symptoms for at least six months.[4] This is to rule out the possibility that what you're experiencing is a sort of blip, rather than a fully established phobia.

A lot more common than full-blown emetophobia is a fear of vomiting. So, if you feel you have difficulties with vomiting, but don't meet the full criteria for emetophobia, this may be the correct diagnosis for you. If this applies to you, I hope many elements of this book will still be helpful. I should warn you, though, that this book contains descriptions of what it is like to experience emetophobia at its worst. Just be aware that you needn't worry – there's nothing to suggest your fear will develop into a phobia. Remember, also, that the symptoms and behaviours of emetophobia that I describe are merely symptoms of an illness and should be viewed as such. What I'm trying to say is, don't take any of them onboard as things you should be concerned by or adopt.

Okay, safety briefing over.

The anxiety

Let's look more closely at some of the primary symptoms of emetophobia. One of the main hallmarks of the condition is anxiety. It's fundamentally an anxiety disorder. While anxiety is a symptom of emetophobia, the anxiety itself can also cause a range of unpleasant and debilitating physical symptoms including:

- nausea
- stomach pain
- a racing heart and/or palpitations
- sweating
- diarrhoea
- breathlessness
- light-headedness
- shaking.

Sound familiar? It certainly does to me! Teenage me was good at shaking. All morning, every morning. Violent, violent shaking. I like to think it counted as some sort of whole-body workout, utilising every muscle until I was as toned as an Olympian.

Not only was I the master of shaking, but I also had nausea down to a tee. Nausea caused by anxiety, caused by a phobia of vomiting. What a mess!

I have many memories of retching behind trees on my way into school, or behind the PE department's hockey-stick-filled pavilion en route to assembly... In fact, almost all my teen memories involve shaking, nausea or a heady combination of the two. Throw in a bit of low-blood-sugar-induced light-headedness and a good old surge of cortisol and you just about have it. Dreamy.

I wasn't alone – in one study, sixty-five percent of people

with emetophobia reported suffering such severe nausea that it interfered with their day-to-day activities, and nearly fifty percent said their nausea was so bad they thought they would be sick.[5]

Isn't it beautifully ironic that one of the main symptoms of a phobia of vomiting is nausea? Let's all take a moment to enjoy that irony... Well done to whatever higher power came up with that hilarious joke. Very funny.

The safety-seeking behaviours

Another almost universal symptom of emetophobia is practising 'safety-seeking behaviours'. But what are they?

Such is their terror, people with emetophobia tend to obsessively engage in activities and behaviours that make them feel safer, or more in control. These actions are their way of trying to reduce their chance of being sick, often very successfully, but sometimes at a very high cost. They include:

- frequently seeking reassurance from others
- obsessively checking how other people are feeling
- looking out for bathrooms and exits in all rooms
- checking food is fully cooked or overcooking food
- refusing to eat foods perceived to be high risk, such as leftovers, shellfish, poultry, bagged salad and food prepared by other people
- eating very small quantities and not eating before going out
- taking anti-nausea medication excessively

- not drinking alcohol
- avoiding children as they tend to be ill more often
- always carrying spare clothes, water and mints
- dodging people who have been unwell
- repeatedly checking use-by dates and food hygiene ratings.

There are endless other examples and every person with emetophobia has their own personal collection of safety-seeking behaviours – kind of like mementoes one collects over time – but these are some of the most common ones.

To reassure you, Dr Alexandra Keyes and Professor David Veale, who have written a book called *Free Yourself from Emetophobia*, say, 'These strategies are completely understandable given how scared you might feel at the thought of vomiting or being around someone who is vomiting. When we are very afraid, it is only natural to want to protect ourselves.'[6]

So, don't beat yourself up about them – the experts say they make sense! But always hold them for what they are – acquaintances that may feel necessary during a difficult journey, not lifelong friends.

The constant fear

Constant fear about vomiting is also a sign of emetophobia. As you've probably gathered by now, people with emetophobia have a completely disproportionate idea of how awful vomiting is, which is why they're so afraid. They view it as catastrophic and believe that the suffering, judgement and embarrassment they would be faced with were they to be sick would be unbearable, hence the desire to avoid it at all costs.

People with the phobia can't deal with the uncertainty of not knowing when, or if, they, or someone around them, might throw up and so will not take any risks.[7] They believe vomiting can happen anywhere and at any time, so live in constant fear.[8] This, really, is the crux of it. Constant fear caused by constant uncertainty. What a way to live!

As part of my research for this book, I spoke to Becky, who has had emetophobia since childhood, and she explained that she is always afraid of encountering vomit. She said she's hypervigilant to the behaviour of others and is always looking out for signs that someone might be sick.

She told me, 'I'm always kind of watching people and wondering if anyone looks like they're ill – it's always there in the background.'

What scares someone with emetophobia more than anything else is human bodies – and there ain't no way of escaping from them, so there's no way of escaping the fear.

Living with emetophobia is like making someone with a phobia of flying take daily long-haul flights on the most turbulent routes, or akin to forcing a person with a terror of spiders to work in the zoo's arachnid house.

It's torture, basically. But you can get better.

As well as constant fear, many people with emetophobia

report repeatedly experiencing intrusive thoughts about being sick. So, for example, if they are sitting on a bus, they might suddenly picture themselves throwing up in the aisle. These unwarranted thoughts and images serve to further increase the worry and anxiety by bringing the thought of vomiting to the forefront of their mind.

The panic attacks

Now that you know all this, it's hardly going to come as a surprise to you that panic attacks are a very common symptom in people with emetophobia. Notably, people with emetophobia tend to report lengthy periods of panic – much longer than panic attacks are conventionally understood to be.[9] That was certainly my experience – when I was a teenager I had panic attacks for hours every morning on school days.

Panic attacks cause symptoms similar to anxiety, but more severe. In addition to the symptoms of anxiety we have already looked at, panic attacks can cause:

- chest pain
- hot flushes or chills
- numbness or pins and needles
- a feeling of impending doom
- derealisation – a feeling of being detached from your body
- a dry mouth or choking sensation.[10]

These episodes of panic are generally triggered by a bodily sensation, such as a momentary stomach cramp or digestive gurgle. Sensations that most people would barely register, and which are harmless, can cause full on panic attacks in people with emetophobia.

They still do in me from time to time.

This is because people with emetophobia tend to be hyper-aware of such sensations and to catastrophise – to view a situation as much worse than it actually is – so, when they register one of these feelings, they assume it means they are going to be sick, and they panic. Someone without the phobia either wouldn't notice the sensation at all or would respond rationally and proportionately and pay no attention to it.

Experts generally agree that emetophobia is one of the most difficult anxiety disorders to live with. It's also surprisingly common and, despite that, there's very little research and help available. Here's to trying to help solve that problem!

Disordered eating

We will cover eating in detail in Chapter 3, so I'll keep it brief for now. People with emetophobia often show signs of disordered eating because they are afraid that food will make them sick. They may fear food poisoning or that over-eating and having too much in their stomach will make them throw up. As a result, they often eat very restrictive diets and practise a lot of rules and rituals around food in a bid to try to reduce their risk of being sick. This disordered eating can cause weight loss, malnutrition and difficulties with work and social life. See Chapter 3 for the full story!

My experience

When I was fully in the grips of emetophobia, the possibility of being sick was a threat that consumed me. It tormented me. It dictated my life. I lived with endless panic attacks and symptoms of anxiety – nausea, shaking, headaches, loss of appetite and faintness – because I was permanently terrified of vomiting.

I didn't trust my body – I viewed it as a feral vessel which I was trapped inside, and judged for, but which I couldn't fully control, and which might let me down catastrophically at any moment. When I put it like that, it does sound rather terrifying! Let's move on rapidly from that thought...

As we've explored, one of the main signs of emetophobia is people going out of their way – a long way out of their way – to avoid the risk of being sick by employing safety-seeking behaviours. They do this in a bid to make themselves feel safer and more in control. It's why people with emetophobia often avoid foreign travel, boats, public toilets, alcohol, hospitals, and some even pregnancy.[11]

As a teenager, I was the master of the safety-seeking behaviours. Or maybe they were the masters of me... I avoided all meals out at restaurants or other people's houses, nights away, holidays, trips to theatres or cinemas, swimming, outings anywhere that didn't have a readily accessible bathroom – such as country walks – and anything that involved driving more than about twenty minutes from home.

Basically, I had no life. I had emetophobia instead. Lucky me!

I wasn't so afraid of reasons for being sick that I felt were 'socially acceptable', such as seasickness, or alcohol-induced vomiting, though unsurprisingly, I was far from keen. These ailments also have the distinct advantage of not being contagious.

In my case, food was the biggest challenge because of the risk of food poisoning. I will come to that topic. Food is a massive one, as I'm sure you know. But when I was chatting to Becky, she said that what she struggles most with is sickness bugs, whereas she's okay with food. So, we are all different.

Becky explained that if someone is travel sick, or sick because they have had a coughing fit, she is okay about looking after them but that what terrifies her is stomach bugs.

She said, 'I get really concerned if I think someone in my family has caught a stomach bug, or if I think one's going to spread and, in particular, if I think I'm going to catch it.'

Becky explained that if anyone in her house is sick, she's excessively careful about cleaning. For example, she said she'll bleach door handles, work surfaces, towels and light switches in a bid to stop the spread of the virus.

I also spoke to Zara, who is twenty and has emetophobia. She told me she's more afraid of other people being sick than of vomiting herself. She explained that the biggest impact the phobia has on her life is that she struggles with social events when people are drinking because she's had so many experiences at university of people getting so drunk they're sick. Same phobia as me, completely different struggles.

However, another example Zara gave was that she recently broke her collarbone falling from a horse and was prescribed codeine for pain relief, but the drug made her sick, so she stopped taking it.

She said, 'I made myself go through the whole recovery with just paracetamol which I found hard, but I would rather feel the pain than be sick.'

To get back to me, I also found foreign travel very difficult. Again, that was really about the food – a fear of foreign food or water making me unwell. I had a misconception that as soon as I left home turf, everything was contaminated by bacteria my body was unused to and which may, therefore, make me ill. Like 'Delhi Belly' but which I thought I risked as soon as I travelled more than fifty miles from home. Never mind Delhi, to me Paris was synonymous with parasites, Barcelona was a hotbed of bacteria, and viruses abounded in Vienna. Only Southeast England felt safe.

Somehow, to me anyway, bacteria in food and water felt more insidious – harder to control and quantify – than travel sickness, morning sickness or alcohol-induced sickness. With the latter, you know exactly why you're being sick, what has caused it and roughly how long it will last. Personally, I find that easier to deal with.

Becky agrees. She said, 'I can deal with my friends being drunk and vomiting. I have many a time held back hair and looked after them while they've been unwell because of alcohol. That doesn't bother me in the slightest because I know I can't catch it, and I know I'm not going to be sick.'

In fact, why is it that someone throwing up because they've downed too many pints is seen as funny, whereas vomiting caused by, say, some dodgy sushi or norovirus is viewed as disgusting?

Public places

People with emetophobia tend to be particularly scared of being sick in public because of the shame they feel it would provoke. This can manifest in behaviours like avoiding crowded theatres and cinemas or always sitting in the seat nearest the door to be able to escape as easily as possible.

For years, when I was a teenager, sitting in a theatre or cinema was close to my idea of hell. Not as close as working in a raw-chicken-processing factory would be, but close enough. School assembly was the same. Agony. I avoided these settings at all costs (I was not averse to legging it down the fire escape to dodge morning assembly).

If I were unlucky enough to find myself trapped in one of these venues, I would be in such a panic I wouldn't absorb a single word of whatever the film, play or lecture was. Many a Shakespeare play in London's West End fell on deaf ears during my English literature course. I'd be completely lost in my own world of torment, aware of nothing other than my panic, all-consuming nausea and desire to run away at top speed. Flight mode in overdrive. Like my primal instincts were reacting to a starving lion flying at my head, rather than to an elderly actor droning on.

Who has it?

We have now, I think, clocked that this thing isn't a bunch of laughs, but how many people have it and who are they?

While most people have never heard of it, emetophobia is surprisingly common. In fact, it's thought to be the most common phobia people seek treatment for,[12] not only because it's common, but, also, because it's so debilitating for those who live with it.

The charity EmetAction reckons the best estimate is that about one in every two hundred people has emetophobia. It believes that about seven percent of the population also has a fear of vomiting, but in a much less severe form than that experienced by people with emetophobia.[13]

The difference is that people who have a fear, as opposed to the full-blown phobia, don't suffer significant distress as a result, and their lives are not negatively impacted.[14] The definition of a phobia is a fear that is 'overwhelming and debilitating'.[15] In other words, if it doesn't completely screw up your life, it's a fear not a phobia.

Emetophobia usually develops in childhood or adolescence, with the average patient starting to show symptoms at the age of just nine.[16] But it can appear at any age. As I've been writing this book it has amazed me how many people have told me they have emetophobia. Until I started talking about it, I'd never heard anyone else mention it. Zara confirmed that this was also her experience. She said she now knows a few people with it and that she gets the impression it is quite widespread, especially among teenage girls.

Certainly, emetophobia is more common in girls and women than boys and men. Estimates vary but ninety percent of sufferers are women, according to one.[17]

But why is emetophobia so much more common in women than men? One theory is that women are more prone to feelings of disgust than men, which makes them more likely to have a problem with sick.[18] It makes sense. From my experience, at least, men are much more likely to be amused by toilet humour, farting and the like. I think we can all picture a couple of men at a sports game laughing at a vulgar joke while the women around them roll their eyes and give them disapproving looks. Just me?

Zoe, a lawyer who has had emetophobia for as long as she can remember, said, 'I can relate to the disgust thing. I can't look at sick. I won't look at it. If I'm sick, I turn all the lights off so I can't see it. I find the idea of stomach contents really disgusting – I see it as vile and disgusting whereas other people seem to find it funny.'

The stats around emetophobia make for bleak reading, especially now we know how many people are living with it. A study found that ninety percent of people with emetophobia are distressed by the condition fifty-two weeks a year and that only twelve percent have experienced a period of more than six months' remission.[19] Come on! Let's bust these stats together!

What causes it?

So, we now know what emetophobia is and who has it. But what causes it? Why did I get it, but my best friend didn't? The unhelpful answer is that no one really knows for sure what causes emetophobia. However, there are various theories and a range of possible factors at play.

Most experts believe that childhood experiences can play a role in the development of this phobia. For example, if a child is made to feel embarrassed or ashamed for being sick this may increase their risk of developing emetophobia in future. Both upsetting experiences of being ill, and of other people's reaction to an illness, can be potential triggers.[20]

However, many people with this phobia remember no such incident. They may, instead, have a memory of being extremely distressed by seeing someone else vomit or become very unwell. Or they may have had no negative experiences of illness at all.[21]

Zara said she doesn't remember a specific trigger event but that her emetophobia emerged when she was about fifteen and started to be exposed to people getting drunk and being sick. She says this was the first time she'd been exposed to people vomiting near her and that it led her to start avoiding situations where she might encounter sick.

Remy, who is a twenty-year-old student, agreed. She told me she's always been upset by being sick but that her emetophobia developed when she was about sixteen without any obvious trigger.

However, Becky does remember a trigger event. She explained she hasn't been sick since she was seven or eight years old and that on that occasion she was being looked after by her brother because her parents were at work.

She said, 'I just remember that it felt really horrible not having my mum there... I felt like the experience of vomiting was horrible and then I also felt quite unsafe.'

Becky went on to explain that because she doesn't tend to catch sick bugs, so has very little experience of vomiting, the notion built up in her mind to be a huge and scary thing.

Becky reflected, 'I think a lot of my issues with emetophobia might stem from a lack of control – I am a bit of a control freak, and I think because this is something I can't control it is problematic for me... I can't control who has stomach bugs or whether people on a plane are ill. Vomiting is a feeling of being out of control.'

Zoe also remembers a trigger event. She told me she remembers her parents once having food poisoning when she was a child and recalls that a friend had to come and look after her and her siblings.

She said, 'My dad is hard as nails, and he never missed work – he never even took a holiday – but he was off this time and that really impacted me. I remember that it was very scary, and I thought that if Dad was off work it must be really bad.'

* * *

So, those are the experiences of some people with emetophobia but there are, of course, other possible factors that can lead to the development of emetophobia. Most people with the phobia probably develop it because of a combination of influences.

Genetics are thought to play a role, specifically a genetic predisposition towards anxiety.[22] So, a person with a close relative who suffers from anxiety, depression or, even, emetophobia itself may be more likely to develop it. Those with a tendency to feel nauseous when anxious can also be more prone to it.[23]

In my case, I know I have a genetic tendency towards developing anxiety – my dad has it, for a start. My mum probably does too, in her own way. It doesn't look good for me, genetically, now I come to think about it!

I'm also a woman – another major risk factor. I believe that these factors, as well as a tendency towards perfectionism and a constant desire for control, make me vulnerable to the development of mental health problems. I know, though, that there was then a specific trigger event, which I will come to, that released the beast.

Maybe it was this specific incident which led to the vulnerabilities in me presenting as emetophobia. I doubt, though, that if that hadn't happened my mental health would have remained fully sound. I suspect, taking my risk factors and personality into account, that if it hadn't presented as emetophobia, it would have come out as a different mental health challenge.

What drives it?

So, what fuels the fire of this phobia? What makes it tick day in, day out? What makes it so powerful? For most people, me included, it's understood to be a vicious cycle that goes like this: Charlie (a stereotypical, but fictional, teenager with emetophobia) feels sick/bloated/has tummy pain and believes this means he will throw up. Charlie then imagines himself vomiting and regards this as a horrific and unmanageable experience. This causes Charlie, who probably isn't good at tolerating the uncertainty that goes hand-in-hand with nausea, to feel anxious. The anxiety causes adrenaline to be released which makes Charlie feel more nauseous and unwell. And so it goes on. Round and round, endlessly.[24]

Understanding this, it makes sense that Charlie will then go out of his way to try to avoid nausea at all costs, pretty much literally. Indeed, many people with emetophobia report they would genuinely rather die than be sick.[25] If vomiting is the most terrifying thing imaginable, then death is preferable.

This avoidance makes the whole problem worse in the long run. For example, Charlie is so scared of feeling sick that he will spend a lot of time thinking about, and planning, how to avoid the risk of vomiting or seeing anyone else vomiting. This makes sense in the short term but actually keeps this emetophobia sufferer focused on the fear which, in turn, keeps the phobia going.[26]

Another trap Charlie may fall into is overanalysing himself and his body for signs of illness. This is a very common behaviour in people with emetophobia but the trouble with it is that, while failing to find any signs may be momentarily reassuring, this inward-looking approach also keeps the mind on the thought of sick, and, yup, you guessed it, feeds (unfortunate choice of word) the phobia.[27]

The more he thinks about it, the more likely he is to feel sick too. In the same way, when I received an email from my children's school this morning saying there was an outbreak of headlice in their class, my head immediately started itching. If you are always thinking about being sick, you're going to feel sick.

Emetophobia experts Dr David Russ and Anna Christie say, 'People with phobias of dogs, clowns, injections, and heights can usually just avoid them. But people with emetophobia cannot avoid their own bodies...often they experience a low level of nausea almost every day, keeping them chronically in a state of anticipation.' They add that this is 'excruciating' and 'no way to live'.[28]

Charlie is also making his problems worse in another way. It's like the opposite of exposure therapy. He avoids things he fears will make him sick. This kind of helps him cope on a day-to-day basis because it makes him feel more in control and safe from the thing he's most afraid of.

However, what he's really achieving is depriving himself of the opportunity to learn that these things are perfectly safe. He's teaching his brain that they're dangerous and need to be avoided. So, in the long run, avoidance behaviours make things worse. They exacerbate the problem because they reinforce the anxiety – they act as a way of telling the anxious voice in his head that there is a real threat and that actions need to be taken to protect himself.

Charlie is far from alone in his use of safety-seeking behaviours. Becky said that she had to take a flight in December and that she'd heard a lot about norovirus on the news, so she wore a face mask on the plane because it made her feel safer. She says she used this safety-seeking behaviour because she was scared of being sick and of the impact that would have on her family's Christmas.

However, were Charlie just to give these things a go, he would, theoretically, learn that they aren't nearly as risky as he believes. If someone is terrified of flying but braves a short flight which goes completely smoothly, they will hopefully be less fearful next time because they had a good experience and have gained confidence in the process. It's the same with people with emetophobia and the things they fear and avoid.

Indeed, were Charlie just to let go a bit and do something that does make him vomit (horror of horrors!), he may just find that it isn't as bad as he suspects.[29] The thought of being sick is a lot worse than the reality for many people with emetophobia, me included. In fact, on the very rare occasions when I have been sick, I've been completely relaxed about it. Where's the sense in that?

Similarly, when Charlie tries to give himself a sense of control by sticking to safety-seeking behaviours, he's worsening the problem by making himself feel like he has some form of control over it and that he needs to exercise it rigorously to keep himself safe. So, whenever he obsessively checks food hygiene ratings, or bleaches the kitchen surfaces into oblivion, he deprives himself of the opportunity to learn that maybe, just maybe, this isn't necessary.[30] Moral of the story? Try it and find out.

The conclusion

In a nutshell, that's what emetophobia is, its symptoms, what causes it and how it takes control. As we go through this book, we will look at many of the ways it can impact people's lives, and at how best to survive while living with it. We will then move on to the ultimate goal of how to recover from it. But first, I will explore in more detail where it comes from and how the phobia developed in me.

Chapter 2

WHERE IT ALL BEGINS

Origins in childhood

Now we know what emetophobia is, let's investigate where it comes from. What triggered it in me? What triggered it in you, for that matter?

As we know, emetophobia most commonly emerges in children and teenagers. This is when it tends to appear in a specific and diagnosable form. However, people who develop the phobia often show a tendency towards anxiety long before their emetophobia presents.

In my case, the emetophobia developed when I was a teenager, but that wasn't when the anxiety started. It started years earlier.

I remember feeling anxious throughout my childhood. I would feel unwell before a school day, get very anxious about people being car sick, and be extremely picky about food. Then there was a spell of obsessive compulsive disorder (OCD) when I was, maybe, eight or ten. But lots of children are fussy about food. Plenty get tummy aches when nervous. None of it was noteworthy at the time, but, looking back, it was a precursor to what was to come...

How my emetophobia started

One night, when I was fourteen, I went to bed a happy, healthy, and rather lazy, teenager. My mind was possessed with no greater concerns than how to get out of the maths homework I didn't understand (because I'd been gossiping all lesson), and whether I could beat my best friend round the school cross-country run without any training.

When I woke up the next morning, I had a debilitating anxiety disorder.

What had happened during that night? As far as I'm aware, absolutely nothing. I'd slept peacefully.

It was just after the Easter holidays. When I woke up, I felt okay, but as the bus neared school I started to feel increasingly unwell – faint, sick and shaky. By the time I got to school, I was white as a sheet, had an upset stomach, and the look in my eyes of a rabbit in headlights.

My teacher took one concerned look at me, assumed I had some nasty, contagious illness, and packed me straight off to the school nurse. Said nurse fed me an apple and told me to lie down on the flimsy, greying sheets of sickbay for half an hour, leaving me no choice but to reluctantly obey.

Rather surprisingly, the apple remedy seemed to do the trick and after an hour or so I returned to lessons, and everything appeared fine.

I was then okay for the rest of the day. It was out of character, though. I was a robust sort of child, had never before visited sickbay, and never missed a moment's school. In fact, I was rather smug about my one hundred percent attendance record and considered myself above the bugs that impacted the mere mortals around me. What a charming teenager I was!

The next morning, I felt sick again and had a sore stomach. I told Mum and let on that the day before I'd spent the morning in sickbay. You see, very unwisely, I tended to keep such things to myself. With this additional information, and the knowledge that I almost never asked to miss school, Mum accepted my case and said I could stay at home.

As a naive, and totally unworldly, fourteen-year-old before the days of Instagram and TikTok, I had no idea that what I was battling was anxiety. I wracked my brain to work out the cause of my nausea. Was it something I'd eaten? A bug? As time went on, those explanations became improbable. Maybe I was allergic to something? Had some horrendous disease?

That it was all in my head never occurred to me.

I spent hours googling 'causes of long-term nausea'. I was quite convinced I had everything from a brain tumour to diabetes. But I never asked anyone for help. I was embarrassed about raising it and so maintained a 'stiff upper lip'. I'd never heard people discuss their mental health. I'm not sure I'd even heard of anxiety. I certainly didn't know what it was or consider that I may be suffering from it... I fear this makes me sound very old. I'm not old – understanding of mental health has just moved on very fast!

So, I was kept off school ill. Vague symptoms. Nausea. Fatigue. Not myself. Generally not feeling well. Uncharacteristically quiet and low in energy.

After about a week, Mum became sufficiently concerned that she took me to the doctor. He said it was nothing and I'd get better soon. But I didn't. So, she took me back. I had blood tests, including one for glandular fever. Everything was normal. Test results were normal. Examination was normal. And yet, I felt no better.

After a couple of weeks and no conclusive test results, the doctor said it was probably anxiety and that I should be sent back to school immediately. And so I was. Shipped back feeling no better than I had on the first day of my illness.

Once it had been deemed to be psychosomatic, it was not considered to be the doctor's problem. No attempt was made to discover what the root of my anxiety might be. I guess everyone assumed it was just a minor blip that was best not given too much attention and that would soon pass. To be honest, that's probably how I would now address a similar situation with my own children, so I'm not criticising. I, also, don't believe in making mountains out of what are probably molehills.

I can only wonder whether things would have worked out differently had it been properly diagnosed and treated at that point. Maybe the condition was still too early in its development to be diagnosable? I think that's probably the case. My sense is that it was more generalised anxiety than fully formed emetophobia.

It's important to point out that this was in the early 2000s, and my doctor was nearing retirement. Basically, he was of a different generation to today's doctors. I hope, and believe, that you will have a very different experience to me. Understanding of mental health has come on such a long way since I was a teenager that doctors now are generally clued up, empathetic and supportive. Don't let my experience put you off seeking the help you need!

At school, it was similar. On my return, I was hauled before my teacher once again and told that I wasn't to worry because all would be well, and she would find a way of solving the problem for me. That was the last I heard from her on the topic.

Again, pastoral support in schools, colleges and universities now is incomparable to when I was at school twenty years ago. As I'm sure you know, they now have well-informed teams perfectly equipped to recognise students who are struggling and to offer them appropriate support. I hope this is your experience!

If not, please don't give up – these institutions have a duty of care and should be held to it. So, speak up, if needs be. Explain what's going on and what support you need. If you aren't able to do so yourself, ask an advocate – maybe a parent – to do it for you. Don't allow yourself to be failed by the system that's meant to help you.

To return to my tale of woe, life went on as normal. For everyone else, that is. The doctor and my teacher forgot about the whole business, and I didn't bother to mention it again. But I felt no better. For the next four years of school, I felt sick. Every day.

It's amazing how quickly abnormal things become normalised – feeling sick soon became my 'normal', and when things are normal, you don't question or address them.

I recollect sitting in the hot, stuffy hall trying to concentrate on my end-of-year exams through wave after wave of debilitating nausea. The room was crammed full of desks and had an unnerving mirror covering the entire end wall for use during dance lessons. At the time I had no idea why I felt so unwell. It would be five years before I found out what was wrong with me, and before I started to feel better.

All I can say is that I hope today's improved access to information and better treatment of mental health means that you get answers more quickly than I did. In fact, I suspect you already have a lot of answers.

The trigger

I have often wondered what triggered the anxiety disorder to develop on that day in the summer term when I was fourteen. It had clearly been simmering under the surface all my life. But why did it choose that day to rear its ugly head? Could I have done something which would have prevented the illness developing?

I suspect puberty and the hormone chaos it causes probably contributed. Maybe the increasing pressure at school as I hurtled towards public exams was also a factor?

But no. Waking up with emetophobia one morning in the summer term wasn't completely out of the blue. I believe I know what triggered it – there was also that event I mentioned earlier.

It was on a family holiday abroad during the Easter break shortly after I turned fourteen. I was with my parents and brothers. Nice hotel, beautiful weather, swimming, right on the beach, walks to local seaside restaurants, and lots of water sports. It was lovely and I was having fun.

But about halfway through the holiday I developed a tummy bug. Nothing particularly dramatic. Just an upset tummy from foreign food and water. It confined me to the hotel room for three days of reading, watching TV and dashing to the loo. It wasn't a big deal at the time. Nonetheless, I think it had a big impact on me emotionally.

It's understood that having a stomach bug at a vulnerable time in a person's life can trigger emetophobia.[1] This seems to have been what happened to me. As a teenager, I was at a vulnerable stage in my development and was, therefore, ill-equipped to handle an illness that would, at other times, have had no lasting impact.

Indeed, I was very sick one afternoon last week for reasons unknown and, while I didn't particularly enjoy the experience,

I really wasn't all that bothered and had fully got over the physical, and psychological, impact within a few days.

So, the point is that my illness came at a bad time. It was embarrassing for a fourteen-year-old. Let's be honest, we're often quite body-conscious or body-self-conscious as teenagers anyway, aren't we? We may be aware of how puberty is causing our bodies to change and of the impact our developing bodies can have on other people. So, maybe, this illness sort of took that natural teenage body focus in me and skewed it in all the wrong ways.

Okay, I'm winging it now. Excuse the pseudo-psychology. I'm not a psychologist. I'm a geographer. I merely dabble in psychology. Dare I say it, it's rather more interesting than atmospheric processes and central business districts. Well, each to their own.

What I do know is how the experience made me feel. It made me feel unsafe and exposed, as though I couldn't rely on my body to behave. I was existing in an unpredictable and unreliable costume that was part of me but was not fully under my conscious control.

That was a huge realisation. If I could get sick on holiday, it could happen any time. What if I was sick at school? That would be embarrassing, wouldn't it? What about when I was out with friends? Or on a daytrip or staying with relatives? Humiliating and awkward. And it could happen suddenly and unexpectedly. Terrifying. I couldn't trust my body.

Right. That's the sanitised version of the story. The U-rated telling. Actually, the E-rated one – Emetophobia Safe. Skip the next few paragraphs if you want to avoid the details. The bit that really did the damage, that caused the trauma that led to the emetophobia.

Okay, so for those brave souls who are joining me in this... actually, it's requiring a fair bit of bravery from me too. It was about twenty years before I could tell this story at all, and then only in writing... This is the full account of what triggered my emetophobia: a couple of days into my illness, I was persuaded to leave the safety of the air-conditioned hotel room and to go and sit by the pool with the rest of the family.

Initially I resisted. Said I wasn't feeling well enough. If only I had stuck to my guns! But I was only fourteen, right? So, I kind of had to do what I was told. And I could see the point that I'd probably be fine just sitting by the pool reading a book and that it would be good for me to get out of the room and try to make the most of the holiday.

As soon as I set foot outside, I knew it was a bad idea. I was immediately hit by a wall of heat and humidity that was too much for my fragile stomach. Nonetheless, I gingerly walked the short distance to the pool where I perched myself on a sun lounger in the shade.

Before I could even open my book, my stomach gave a series of ominous gurgles, and I knew I needed to get to the loo and sharpish. I marched at top speed back towards the safety of my room. As I crossed the wide, sun-drenched stretch of lawn in front of our block I had an accident.

Having just read that bit back, I feel like running rapidly back to the E-rated bit too. In fact, I'm going to ask my husband, Jamie, whether people without emetophobia would view that story as perfectly acceptable or falling into the TMI category. I simply don't know – my perception of these things is too skewed.

Anyway, that's when my anxiety disorder began. Suddenly I felt unsafe and vulnerable and scared all the time because I was always in my body, and yet I had lost faith in it. It was an out-of-control being that I had to do everything possible to maintain control of. I could never be safe again because I could never escape from the risk.

I guess what I really wanted was for my mind to be able to exist without my body. I realise now that this sounds like some sort of death wish, but I wanted to be free of all physical confines, and certainly of all bodily processes. I wanted the purity of just a mind, one that didn't require mucky things like food and didn't go to the loo or get sick or sneeze or cough or burp. It strikes me now how deeply ironic this desire was given that it was my mind causing all my troubles. I craved cleanliness and purity and simplicity. Those things, perfection and control.

I should also say that this was a slightly unusual emetophobia trigger in that it didn't involve vomiting – I'm possibly a slightly atypical case because I have as much fear of diarrhoea (wow, that word is hard to spell! Best to resort to my friend's spelling – dire rear) as vomiting. It all amounts to much the same thing, though, so don't write me off here!

The power of the gut microbiome

Another theory about how this illness on holiday triggered my emetophobia has also dawned on me recently. It was even confirmed by a therapist as possibly having some legs.

There's increasing understanding in medical circles of the power of the gut microbiome – namely, the trillions of little bugs that live in our guts – over our mental health and well-being. It's also generally accepted that having a stomach bug can cause changes to a person's gut microbiome. So, it's just possible that this illness I had may have caused a big enough change of guard among my gut bugs to alter the chemical messages being sent to my brain and, thereby, to have shifted my thinking from a largely healthy pattern to an anxious one.

As my gut microbiome wasn't tested before, or after, the illness we will never know but as doctor and popular podcaster, Dr Rangan Chatterjee, confirms, 'It's becoming clear that the importance to our mental and physical health of having a healthy microbiome can hardly be overstated.'[2]

He adds, 'These trillions of bacteria interact with each other, and with us, and have huge impacts on our health. Their make-up and diversity influence everything from our gut function to our mood.'[3]

So, to put it crudely, is it possible that the gut microbiome I had prior to that illness was one that produced all the chemicals I needed for good health, whereas the one I was left with afterwards didn't? Or, at least, that the changes were sufficient to push my emotional state over the threshold between healthy and unhealthy?

Trauma

What I want to understand now is why it took two or three weeks for the anxiety disorder to appear after this event. Why did it not appear immediately after that trauma? What internal, or subconscious, processes were going on in that time? Could anything have been done in that window to prevent the emetophobia developing?

In a bid to get to the bottom of this, I'm going to consult the work of trauma expert, Dr Bessel van der Kolk. Dr van der Kolk says that trauma robs people of the feeling that they're in charge of themselves; that it can make people behave as though they're constantly at risk of catastrophe. He says that when people experience a traumatic event, such as my illness on holiday, it can make them overreact to other, ordinary, events in life.[4] Yes! Thank you, Dr van der Kolk. That's spot on!

Another example of this would be that my husband, Jamie, witnessed our daughter's traumatic birth and near death and, as a result, now panics at the slightest sign of illness in the children or hint of danger, such as tree climbing. As he puts it, Sophie's birth taught him that sometimes planes really do crash – no one expects their child to be life-threateningly unwell, but that's what happened to us.

It makes sense with Jamie – Sophie really did come extremely close to death in front of his eyes, and doctors really were desperately battling against the odds to save her life. But why did I get 'traumatised' by something so insignificant?

Let's consult Dr van der Kolk again. He says that if you go through a difficult experience and someone offers to help and support you – if they empathise and talk it through with you – this can be protective and helps you to feel safe again. In other words, it helps to prevent trauma.[5]

Did I feel supported afterwards? Was there anyone around me who walked beside me through that experience? No! I mean, look, to the outside observer it wasn't a big deal anyway. So why would anyone have thought I needed that support? And, also, it was embarrassing. I wasn't going to talk about it! I just wanted to bury my head in the sand and forget the whole thing.

So, as Dr van der Kolk says, after a traumatic experience, people require the support and empathy of loved ones. If they don't receive that, they are at much greater risk of becoming traumatised by the event and suffering adverse impacts on their life as a result. Does this ring true for any trigger event you experienced?

I wonder whether that means that, possibly, during that short window between the trauma and the anxiety disorder developing in me, with the right support, this whole business could have been prevented? I always assumed there was nothing I, or anyone else, could have done at any point to stop me becoming like that.

There's no way of knowing for sure, I know that. But if Dr van der Kolk is right then it seems I must accept that had I felt able to talk openly about that experience, and how upsetting it was, and had someone listened, and empathised, and offered unconditional love and support, it's possible that, maybe, this emetophobia could have been prevented. But we will never know. I'm not sure I knew how harmful that illness had been initially.

It seems to me that this comes down to social conditioning again – were these topics less of a taboo then maybe I would have talked more freely about it, it would have felt less traumatic, and I either wouldn't have needed empathy, or would have accessed it more easily.

The thing to take away from this, though, is that it's always wise to talk to someone you trust and feel comfortable with if you go through an upsetting experience. Bottling things up doesn't tend to end well!

The conclusion

So that is the story of my emetophobia, how it developed, and what triggered it. Of course, everyone's experience is different and not everyone with the phobia recollects any traumatic event at all. Maybe you can also identify the factors that came together to trigger the development of your emetophobia?

Anyway, regardless of how it came about, there are challenges in day-to-day life almost universal to people with emetophobia and it is to those that we will now turn. We will start with the huge, and crucial, issue of food. Buckle up. Let's do this thing...

Chapter 3

THE F WORD

Food. Right. For me, at least, this was the biggest issue caused by emetophobia. It's a complex subject fraught with numerous inconsistencies and challenges. In this chapter, I will do my best to unpick the whole muddle and try to offer some practical tips for eating with emetophobia.

Before we begin, I want to clarify something – I think we can all agree that we don't want just to exist with emetophobia. We don't want always to have our food decisions dictated by this condition, right? The aim is to look at food without an emetophobic lens. In Chapter 7, we will explore how to get to that point – how to overcome the emetophobia for good.

This chapter, though, will deal with the food issues emetophobia can cause and how best to manage with those issues while working towards recovery.

To be clear, I don't want to advocate avoiding foods that make you anxious because, in doing so, you perpetuate the fear. However, I do want to address how you can continue to nourish your body sufficiently for good health while in the grips of this phobia. It's a tricky line to tread.

Eating with emetophobia

Let's look at the deal with food. People with emetophobia, it's well understood, are sometimes so scared of being sick that they will restrict the amount, or types, of food they'll eat. This can lead to malnutrition and to being underweight.[1]

That's certainly what happened to me. In my experience, the problem is twofold. The first element is simple – I couldn't eat because I felt sick.

No one wants to eat when they feel very nauseous or panicky, do they? As a teenager, I was so anxious that my stomach was always churning. So, I never felt able to eat.

Imagine if you were about to give an important presentation in front of your whole school and were very nervous. Would you want to eat a hearty meal at that moment? No, of course not. Well, I felt like that all the time. So, I never felt like eating. If I tried, I would feel like I was going to throw up.

The second factor was more complex and more fundamental. Even if I could, physically, have eaten, I still couldn't have managed it. It's to do with safety and control as, in fact, is everything related to emetophobia, don't you think?

I could only eat foods I considered to be 'safe'; namely, foods I believed least likely to cause food poisoning. And the worse my anxiety, the shorter the list of 'safe' foods became. Moving more foods onto my 'safe list' is something I'm still working on. These days, the list is long and nutritious. When I was in the last couple of years of school, it was extremely short and not at all nutritious.

I guess everyone sticks to a list of safe foods, don't they? I mean, no one eats random, poisonous, red berries from suspect bushes. The problem with emetophobia is that it skews your perception of what should be on the safe list. It can make foods that are perfectly harmless seem too threatening to consume. The more extreme that skewing becomes, the greater the problem.

Food rules

People with emetophobia tend to make food decisions based on a set of food rules – these rules dictate what does, and doesn't, make the safe list.

For example, as a teenager, I couldn't eat meat, fish or raw veg – not safe (oh, sorry – they are, of course, safe really...). Whereas bread with butter, plain pasta, and things in packets, like biscuits or chocolate, were okay. I also needed to know how my food had been stored and prepared – I liked to have control over it, so I knew if it was 'safe'. As a result, I couldn't eat anything prepared by anyone else, or rather, felt I couldn't. I had to make it myself, in a way I was happy with.

But where on earth did all these rules come from? Which foods make a person's 'unsafe' list tends to be driven by things they have seen, heard or read about.[2] So, for example, if someone with emetophobia hears that a friend got food poisoning from sushi, they may stop eating sushi. Or if they read that there is an outbreak of E. coli linked to unpasteurised cheese, they may refuse to eat any unpasteurised dairy products from then on.

It's interesting for me to reflect on where I got my specific set of rules from. Jamie has observed that he thinks a tendency towards scrolling tabloid news websites may be relevant. He pointed out that I actively look for food scare stories and then adapt my behaviour based on what I've read. He's right about that, though it hadn't occurred to me until he said it.

I think my mum would observe that food technology lessons at school also contributed to my list of food rules. There were lessons on food safety, and I suspect I took the food hygiene rules we learned to heart and applied them in an extreme form. For example, I remember being taught that food shouldn't be left out of the fridge for too long. I think we were told that two hours was the safe maximum time. However, in my mind that rule became distorted and twisted to the point at which I wouldn't eat anything that had been out of the fridge for more than about fifteen minutes.

Maybe you can identify food rules you practise? This is a worthwhile exercise because once you know what behaviours you exercise around food, you can start to work through which are logical and reasonable, and which need challenging. It might be an idea to discuss your list with someone you trust and ask them to help you establish which rules are necessary, and which are emetophobia-driven.

Remy told me she won't eat out anywhere unless she's

checked all the restaurant's reviews for any mention of it causing food poisoning. She said she also won't eat anywhere that has fewer than five positive reviews because she needs evidence that it's safe. She said this was particularly challenging when she was travelling around South America on her gap year. She felt she had to scrutinise reviews of every cafe or bar before she could eat there and, even then, while her friends were relaxed, she would obsessively avoid what she considered high-risk foods.

Remy added that sometimes, especially if she's stressed or emotional, the texture of some foods, such as eggs and butter, can make her retch. She said that once a meal has triggered that response, however hungry she is, she can't eat any more of it and feels she must throw it away and get something else to eat.

Zoe also struggles with eating out. She said, 'I love food, but I think carefully about what I choose and if there's something that spooks me about a restaurant, such as that it's empty, I won't eat there. It's like I'm always doing risk assessments. It's exhausting, that hypervigilance – it's a stressful experience.'

Zoe added that she doesn't eat chicken, fried rice or seafood and she checks hygiene ratings carefully before she eats out. She said, 'Recently I ate half a prawn, and I felt like an absolute rebel!'

* * *

I know that my relationship with food was ridiculous in most people's eyes, and that these anxieties were completely out of proportion to the risk. But I didn't know how to conquer them. They were more powerful than my rational brain. I just couldn't override them a lot of the time, or give up the rules. I'm also not entirely sure I wanted to overcome them. They were my safety net. Why would I want to lose behaviours that I'd put in place to keep myself safe?

For me, the idea of not having these rules was like jumping out of a plane without a parachute. Why would I do that? Sound familiar?

What I've realised recently is that I've followed my own safety rules for so long that I no longer know where the healthy or 'normal' line falls. So, for example, I know that no one in their right mind would eat a raw chicken, but that they would eat a properly cooked roast chicken from a reputable butcher or supermarket. Okay. That's easy enough. But where's the line?

Do people who don't have emetophobia eat chicken from dodgy-looking fried chicken shops with poor food hygiene ratings on inner city highways? Some must or those shops would go bust. Or what about chicken curry from street food stalls in India? I don't know.

* * *

When I think about my challenges with food it makes me wonder about anorexia. People with anorexia will literally starve themselves to death because their fear of weight gain is so severe, and their food rules are so strict. If that's possible, maybe it's not so unbelievable that I found eating so hard. Maybe emetophobia isn't that different. It's just a different underlying fear that leads to the difficulties with food.

Dr David Russ and Anna Christie say: 'Emetophobia can be confused with an eating disorder because patients can be anorexic, as "anorexia" literally means "lack or loss of appetite for food"...people with emetophobia may be underweight, have nutritional problems, or display intense control over food.'[3]

Then they go on to explain that anorexia differs from emetophobia in that to be diagnosed with anorexia a person must be obsessed with weight gain and must also have a distorted perception of their own weight, in other words, believe they are overweight when it's clear to everyone else that they are, in fact, underweight.[4] These two factors do not apply in emetophobia.

* * *

When I was in my final year of school, and my emetophobia was at its worst, there were a lot of days when I couldn't eat anything. On those days, nothing felt safe or complied with the rules. I went into the kitchen and looked for something because I knew I needed to eat; I paced around supermarkets looking for anything I could have and could find nothing. I could find not one thing that my anxious brain would let me consume.

I could only imagine the luxury of being able to go to a friend's house for a meal and happily eat whatever I was offered. Or of going to a restaurant and feeling relaxed about choosing and eating whatever I fancied from the menu.

I missed out as a teenager as a result. I couldn't join my friends at dinners. Nor could I go with them on the school ski trip during the Christmas holidays. I couldn't even join them on nights out.

That's an upsetting thought. However, as the psychiatrists say, it really isn't a person's fault if they develop emetophobia – you have no control over your childhood experiences or your genes.[5]

Nonetheless, when I went to a party and watched everyone else effortlessly helping themselves to mounds of tasty morsels from the buffet, I cursed myself for not being able to do the same.

Do other people not look at food and immediately wonder if it might make them ill? It always looked delicious, and I wanted to look after and nourish my body but, even if I was starving, I could take nothing more than some bland bread and butter. It was like the rest wasn't edible in my mind.

Becky empathised. She said if she goes to a BBQ, unless her husband is cooking, she tends to avoid chicken and would very carefully study the food to make sure it's fully cooked. She said she was recently at a BBQ and, even though she enjoys the flavour of seafood, the emetophobic voice in her head wouldn't allow her to have any.

She said, 'It does affect my food choices, and I get nervous when I don't know what other people's food hygiene is like so if we are going to someone's house, I will be careful what

I choose. I tend to stick with things that I know can't give me any sort of stomach upset.'

Becky added that she throws out food as soon as it is past its best before date. She said she also asks her husband to smell meat before cooking it and that she throws it away if it doesn't quite smell right, or if she thinks it doesn't.

Food anxiety and rituals

Now, that was how the food thing worked for me – it was all about the risk of food poisoning. There are, though, other aspects to food anxiety for some people with emetophobia. For example, some only eat very small quantities for fear that if they get too full, they might be sick, or in a bid to ensure that if they are sick there isn't much in their stomach to expunge.[6] Others don't eat for hours before going in a car or on a boat, because they fear it will increase their risk of travel sickness.

I also didn't eat anything I considered remotely 'risky' before going out in case it made me ill when I was out. I would, for example, only eat a cheese and pickle sandwich and an apple at lunch if I were going out in the afternoon, whereas if I was going to be at home in the afternoon, I might have something marginally more exotic.

It's also common for people with emetophobia to practise compulsions or rituals around eating to make themselves feel safer. For example, they may only eat at certain times of day, or in a specific place, or from a particular plate. These compulsions can develop if a person, say, usually eats with the same fork and hasn't been sick after eating with that utensil. They may begin to see it as a sort of lucky charm and fear that, were they to use a different fork, they would be putting themselves at greater risk.

In extreme circumstances, people with emetophobia can even get into a dangerous vicious cycle in which they stop eating altogether.[7] This usually starts with the person with emetophobia experiencing a sensation, such as bloating, which makes them afraid they will be sick. This, in turn, causes them to eat less, which makes their stomach rumble with hunger. They then misinterpret this sensation as nausea, which leads to a further reduction in food intake. This can become a rapid and dangerous downward spiral in which their body starts to shut down from lack of nutrition, leaving them isolating themselves at home in a state of hunger, adrenaline and cortisol-induced terror. The only solution is to eat.

Why you need to address your relationship with food

I know that extending your food repertoire while battling emetophobia is not easy. In fact, I know it can feel virtually impossible. I also know that you can be reluctant to try to do so for fear of the consequences. The whole jumping out of a plane without a parachute thing.

So why bother trying? What's the motivation? Because, the thing is, that when you need to do something that's hard, it's crucial to be clear why you're doing it. You need to be fully committed to the reason or resolve will soon weaken.

As far as I can see, there are four reasons why you need to try:

1. Not eating enough nutritious food is bad for your health and wellbeing both in the short term, and in the longer term.
2. Being malnourished can make emetophobia recovery harder.
3. It's hard to maintain a fully functioning and enjoyable social life while living with very strict food rules.
4. No one wants their life, and their decisions, dictated by an anxiety disorder – it's much more fun just to be able to eat whatever the hell looks most delicious.

Malnutrition

So, what does happen if you don't eat enough, or if you don't get sufficient nutrients? Most people with emetophobia can probably get sufficient calories from their 'safe' foods and eating times, but eating only Mars bars and fries, and only after 8pm, isn't a recipe for good health.

So, it isn't just about eating enough and not being underweight – it's about getting enough nutrients. I did my best to survive on Jaffa Cakes in my last year of school. I lived to tell the tale, but I wouldn't recommend it.

So, the most obvious risk of not eating enough nutritious

food is that of becoming underweight. It's generally recognised that a person is underweight if they have a BMI of less than 18.5. But what on earth is BMI? Well, it's short for Body Mass Index and is calculated by dividing an adult's weight in kilograms by their height in metres squared.[8] Don't panic, though. No need to do any maths – just google it. There are loads of BMI calculators online – just punch in your weight and height and they'll tell you your BMI.

When I was a teenager, and was underweight, my doctor was endlessly telling me that I would get osteoporosis because being too thin meant I wasn't laying down the amount of bone required to avoid the condition as I aged. So, in my mind, that's the main risk.

But let's look at the facts. Being underweight, or not taking in sufficiently nutritious food, can lead to malnutrition. I think many people only associate malnutrition, say, with famines and so think it isn't relevant to them. This isn't true. Malnutrition is simply caused by having low levels of vitamins and minerals in your diet. It's even possible to be overweight and malnourished. This is because you can put on weight just eating, for example, fast food, but it doesn't contain the nutrients required to avoid malnutrition.

Malnutrition[9] can result in:

- a weakened immune system, which puts you at risk of infections and repeatedly catching colds and other viruses
- slow wound healing

- general feelings of weakness
- fatigue
- poor concentration
- depression
- feeling cold all the time
- anaemia
- weak hair and nails.

In women, being underweight and/or malnourished can also lead to fertility issues and can cause your periods to become erratic, or to stop altogether. In your teen years, it can cause problems with growth and development.[10]

Ironically, having a poor diet can also increase the risk, or severity, of mental health problems. It's a sort of vicious cycle – someone doesn't eat well because they have emetophobia, so they aren't taking in the vitamins and nutrients their body needs to thrive, which causes their mental wellbeing to deteriorate further, which makes their anxiety worse – and so it goes on.

So that's why it is important for health to eat well. Don't panic, though. The human body is extremely resilient and can cope with far from ideal nutrition for a long time. So, even if your diet is currently very limited, stay calm and don't fret. Just do your best to start improving it step by step. We aren't aiming for perfection here – we're going for 'good enough'. Even just adding slightly more calories, or a slightly wider variety of foods, will have a positive impact. All you can do is to do your best and to seek the help that is available.

Being malnourished and underweight can also make it harder to recover from emetophobia. When your body is in this state your thinking can become very rigid, and with rigid thinking, emetophobia treatment and recovery is far more difficult.[11]

You see, it's an evolutionary thing: when someone is starving, their brain adapts to be hyper-focused on one thing, and mental flexibility, the ability to switch between perspectives and to see the bigger picture, is lost.[12] For a caveman this would've been helpful because it would've allowed them to harness all their brain power to help them source food. In this case it would potentially have saved them from starving. At times of food shortage, they didn't need to be wasting any mental energy on fighting neighbouring cavemen or drawing pictures of animals on the cave walls – they just needed to focus on finding food to survive.

However, nowadays it can be an unhelpful adaptation. It can mean that your mind becomes completely focused on your emetophobia and you are unable to engage with the ideas and thoughts of others. If you can't accept, or attend to, the possibility of other ways of acting and thinking, you can't get better.

In some cases, nutritional supplements may be needed to help shift your thinking pattern enough to enable you to engage productively with treatment.[13]

Let's now look at the social motivation to improve your eating habits. We will cover this more in the next chapter so let's keep this brief for now...

Social events and eating

It's worth trying to improve your relationship with food because it makes social events easier and more enjoyable. Think about it for a sec. How many social events involve food in one way or another? Brunches, lunches, dinners, take-aways, BBQs, buffets, you know the score. All I'll say about this for now is that it's much easier socially if you can happily just accept these kinds of invitations and eat something when you get there.

None of us wants to draw attention to ourselves by sitting in the corner with an empty plate while everyone else gorges, do we? We don't need to eat piles and piles of buffet offerings. We just need to eat a decent enough range of foods to avoid looks or comments. That's all.

Food freedom

We've established that it's probably worth working on our eating to give ourselves choice and freedom. Thing is, while in the short-term keeping hold of our safety-seeking behaviours might be comforting, and make us feel safer, it's liberating to be able to make food choices based on something other than the risk of being sick – much better to be able to choose based on what looks tastiest, what's most nutritious, or even what is most budget-friendly.

My top tips for eating with emetophobia

Right, time to get to the important bit. As I said, we aren't yet going to tackle how to escape emetophobic thinking around food but let's look at how to maintain a sufficiently nutritious diet until we have escaped emetophobic thinking.

Here are my top tips:

- Make the most of all occasions when you feel able to eat. So, if you have a quiet day at home and are feeling relatively relaxed without the pressure of having to go out, don't spend the entire day doom scrolling or Netflix binging – prioritise packing in the best meals you can manage with some nutritious snacks in between for good measure. In other words, make up for days when you've been busy and felt less able to eat.

- Plan your food for the day in advance. So, for example, if you're going to be out all day, don't leave home in a mad rush thinking you'll grab lunch on the go if you know you won't actually do that. Take something 'safe' with you (I like peanut butter sandwiches, a piece of fruit and some nuts and dried fruit in these circumstances). That way, you'll have something nutritious to have while you're out and you won't end up skipping lunch or eating junk.

- Even if it's repetitive, make the most of the foods you're comfortable eating. Pasta with tomato sauce every night is a whole lot better than nothing, but maybe challenge yourself and add some simple veg on the side.

- Be kind to yourself. Be gentle. Respect that you find eating hard in certain circumstances currently. So, find ways to make as many meals work as possible. For example, if you don't like eating before travelling, get up a few minutes early and make breakfast to take with you to eat when you arrive at school/work/college. Or if you're going out for dinner but know you'll only eat the bread, have something before you go. What works for each person is different depending on exactly what makes them anxious around eating. But be mindful of the problem and try to work around it as well as you can. A bit of honest forethought can go a long way.

- If you don't like to feel full, make sure that every mouthful you eat counts and is as nutritious as possible. Much better to have a few nuts than a few jellybeans, for example. Pack in those nutrients whenever you can!

- Have always to hand – in your kitchen, bag, on your desk, wherever – a selection of nutritious and 'safe' foods for moments of need. Cereal bars, nuts, dried fruit, dark chocolate, fruit, that sort of thing. This means you're never scrabbling around trying to find something to eat at the last minute – as, if you're anything like I was, that won't go well.

- If there are certain foods you don't like to be around, say, raw chicken, then either don't have any in your house or ask your housemates to leave one fridge shelf, chopping board and so on chicken-free so that you never get put off your food by the thought of contamination. I reached a compromise with Jamie where we'd have chicken in the house but only ready-cooked chicken, so there was never raw chicken around, but he could still add a chicken breast to his salad at lunch if he so desired.

- Try to be open and honest about what you will and won't eat if you are going out to dinner with other people. I found this hard, because I didn't like to seem fussy or difficult. I told myself that I'd wing it when I got there, even though I knew perfectly well that I wouldn't. However, it's much better to be honest than to leave the food someone has made for you. So, for example, if you are going to a friend's house for dinner, let them know in advance that you don't eat X, Y or Z (say, chicken and seafood). I often found it easier to say that I was a vegetarian. That wasn't strictly true, but I usually found vegetarian options less threatening. Obviously, it's probably not a good idea to present your unsuspecting hosts with a huge list of banned foods and cooking rules but some simple guidance is often wise.

Our end goal is to overcome emetophobic thinking about food and to not require these tips, but in the meantime, I hope they help you to get the nutrition you need.

So, that's the long and the short of emetophobia and food. It's a huge topic, which impacts each person with the phobia differently, but I hope this chapter has been useful regardless of your specific relationship with food. Let's now move on to look at how to maintain strong friendships, and to keep having FUN, while living with emetophobia, because that's what life is all about really, isn't it?

Chapter 4

RELATIONSHIPS, SOCIAL LIFE AND OPENING UP

Having close friends, good relationships with family and an enjoyable social life is crucial to mental wellbeing and a good quality of life. These things are, therefore, also critical to thriving with, and recovering from, emetophobia. However, living with emetophobia can make maintaining relationships and a fulfilling social life difficult.

This is the challenge we're going to address in this chapter.

Friends

The first question is: how does emetophobia impact people's relationships and social life? Of course, that varies from one person with emetophobia to the next, but the condition can make people avoid any situation they perceive as risky. The trouble with this is that many people with the phobia will avoid risk even if that means cancelling plans at the last minute if they think there's a threat.[1]

If nothing else, repeatedly bailing on your friends doesn't tend to be a good way to maintain relationships, does it? Nor does turning down social invitations because they involve going out of your comfort zone. Friends and colleagues can get the wrong end of the stick and start to take it personally. You know, if your college mates keep inviting you to grab a drink with them at the weekend and you always say no, well, let's be honest, they're going to stop asking after a while, aren't they? They'd be forgiven for thinking you're the busiest person on Earth, or that you just don't want to spend time with them.

Before we look at how to avoid this problem, let's make a list of some more ways in which emetophobia can screw up people's social lives:

- It makes you want to avoid any event involving food.
- It puts you off going into cinemas and theatres.
- It makes you feel anxious about leaving the house.
- It causes nausea and anxiety, which stop anything you do being fun.
- It makes you anxious about intimacy in case you're sick.
- It puts you off the idea of kissing, or other closeness with a partner, in case they are ill, and you catch a bug that makes you sick.
- It makes you want to keep away from people when there are sickness bugs going around.
- It stops you drinking or being around people who are drunk for fear of alcohol-induced vomiting.
- It makes you so constantly focused on the thought of being sick that you can't concentrate on conversations or be emotionally present at social events.

Of course, these are just examples and don't all apply to everyone with emetophobia. There are also plenty of other ways in which the phobia can impact people's social lives. Really, what it boils down to is that for people with emetophobia, avoiding vomit is the most important thing in life and it trumps friendships and relationships at every turn.

Becky said, 'I get scared and quite annoyed if I hear about someone coming to a social gathering when they've been sick the night before – I like people to follow the forty-eight-hour rule and people don't follow that and I find that very scary and inconsiderate.'

She continued, 'I will keep away from anyone who has been sick and if I hear someone has thrown up in the toilets, I won't use them and will wait until I get home. I also make sure I wash my hands carefully and it plays on my mind until enough time has passed that I'm happy I haven't come down with it.'

She explained that all her best friends know about her phobia and are respectful of it, not coming near her if they've been ill. She said she really appreciates this, but that other people aren't always as considerate.

Becky added, 'I absolutely hate winter and norovirus. If I see on the news that there's a big norovirus outbreak, I would rather avoid meeting up with people socially, especially those who have children – I'd rather be at home in a protective bubble. I really find it hard.'

I'm going to be honest. When I was a teenager, I basically

didn't have a social or romantic life because my emetophobia didn't allow it. I did have close friends, but I only really hung out with them when I couldn't get out of it, namely, at school.

As well as a large handful of lovely school friends, I had a best friend to whom I was extremely close. She was crucial to my life at the time, and I hugely valued the closeness we had. While I felt alone with my own head, I never felt alone or lonely on a social level and I'm very grateful for that. Those friendships were part of what enabled me to keep dragging myself into school every day – I knew I had allies at school and that made me feel safer. We also had plenty of side-splitting laughter, usually caused by some gentle misbehaviour in lessons, and laughing always makes you feel better.

Except during our occasional explosive bust-ups, I loved hanging out with my best friend and got a huge amount from the feeling of camaraderie and companionship she offered. She was familiar with anxiety and so seemed to understand my situation, to an extent. She also offered both tough love and empathy, which were helpful in equal measure.

I did see her outside school – I recollect plenty of cups of tea (I don't even like tea so I've no idea why it was always tea) in her parents' kitchen and I think there was even the odd shopping trip to London. Anything more than that, though, was off the cards for me at the time and the outings we did go on were fraught with anxiety and nausea so were never as fun for me as they should have been.

I very rarely went to clubs or pubs or bars or restaurants.

Nor did I have any romantic relationships. A combination of anxiety, nausea and my obsession with getting perfect grades made that impossible... Those and being at an all-girls' school in the middle of a wood... When I got to university, however, I made up for it. But we will come to that later. I missed out on a huge amount of 'normal' teenage experience as a result – I sort of bypassed that part of life and of development – and I want to help you avoid doing the same.

When I was a teenager, every time I contemplated going out with my friends I would immediately think, 'But what if I'm sick?' And then I wouldn't want to go, to avoid the possibility of puking in public. I knew, also, that if I did go, I wouldn't enjoy it because I would be too anxious and feel too sick. So, I stayed at home and did schoolwork instead.

I wasn't unique in having my social life wrecked by emetophobia. Zara told me her social life at university is being impacted by her emetophobia because so often people at parties drink too much and are sick.

She said, 'I avoid the busiest nights out when everyone drinks loads and throws up. I wish I could go – it has held me back socially – but it frustrates me when others don't know their limits. It ends the night for me when someone is sick.'

Becky said, 'I remember when my housemate got a stomach bug, I felt so terrified. I literally remember hiding myself away in my room and as much as possible not coming out and having no contact with her. I almost had the covers of my bed over my head because of the fear that I might catch that stomach bug.'

She added, 'I internalise a lot of the fear because I think people think I'm stupid or irrational. It can make me feel quite panicky, scared and vulnerable. I don't think people who aren't affected by it know how much it plays on your mind in so many ways.'

* * *

However you manage it, it's vital to maintain as many friendships as you possibly can because something as simple as having a cup of tea with a mate, or receiving a friendly message, can give you a real boost, can make you feel happier and can reduce your stress levels.[2]

So, the mere act of having strong relationships can help with managing and overcoming your emetophobia. Humans are fundamentally social animals and do best when they feel part of a tribe. Social isolation and loneliness are also major sources of stress and are very damaging to wellbeing. As a result, the better your relationships, the lower your stress levels, and the greater your happiness. The happier and more relaxed you are, the better placed you will be to tackle your emetophobia. Even if it's hard, it's well worth prioritising social connection. Undoubtedly, I always benefitted from a heart to heart with my best friend at school.

You get the idea: relationships and connection with other people are important. So, what can we do about it?

Communicating

Well, communication is key, but it's thought that a lot of people with emetophobia keep their condition a secret.[3] Does that apply to you? That's a question worth asking yourself and reflecting on because it's something you may want to address.

It seems most people muddle along as best they can without sharing their feelings and anxieties. But why? From my experience, initially at least, this can be because they don't know or understand what on earth is wrong with them or how to explain it. Later it becomes about embarrassment, a fear of being misunderstood or a fear of judgement. Some people are also just inherently quite private and don't feel comfortable talking about their worries and anxieties.

Zara said, 'It can be a difficult thing to explain to people who don't understand. People think it's a weird thing to have a phobia of – they are confused by it and find it random.' Happily, she added that, even if confused, people have always been kind to her about it whenever she's mentioned it.

Even if it doesn't come naturally, I would encourage you to talk about your struggles as much as you can, with people you are close to. The more you share (within reason) the better placed your family, friends, teachers and colleagues will be to understand and support you and the less alone you will feel.

Also, the more you talk about something, the less powerful it often becomes. Like the cliché that a problem shared is a problem halved. If you can talk about it light-heartedly, and see the funny side, so much the better. To employ another cliché, laughter is the best medicine, as long as it doesn't go so far as to downplay the genuine suffering emetophobia causes.

Obviously, don't go on about it ceaselessly until everyone is sick of the topic (pun not intended) – it's about balance, isn't it? You will know where the line of healthy moderation lies. Talk about it enough to explain your feelings, and what you're going through, to your closest friends and family at the right moments. Probably not when you're late for school, the phone's ringing and there's a delivery driver at the door... But don't overdo it.

I know telling someone about your emetophobia for the first time can be difficult and nerve-wracking. If you are worried about it, or afraid you might not be able to explain clearly in the moment, you could try writing down what you want to say – you could have some notes with prompts to help you with the conversation, or you could tell them in writing. Another option could be to send them a voice note – that way you don't have to tell them in person, and you can always delete and re-record the message if you aren't happy with it. These options would also give the person you're telling a chance to pause and come up with a considered response, so it might be easier for them too.

Also, try not always to hide behind a mask either of humour or of stoicism. Of course, those masks have their place and are important in many circumstances. For example, in job interviews or exams there may be something to be said for employing a front of capability, competence and composure...

Not that your emetophobia prevents you being those things as well as emetophobic...

But, in safe moments, with empathetic people, you could experiment with dropping the mask and allowing yourself to be vulnerable. See what happens. My experience is that when you do, it often leads to beautiful and nurturing interactions that can make you feel much closer and more bonded to the friend or relative you're with. That feeling is profoundly relaxing and comforting.

I chatted with Ellie who is seventeen and a student. She developed emetophobia at the age of fifteen after suffering from heat stroke during the school summer holidays. She said she stopped going out with her friends and that as a result they began to think they had done something to upset her, so she explained about her emetophobia.

Ellie said: 'Once they understood, they were happy just to chill at someone's house because they knew I was happier with that. You just have to talk about it and to explain. I'd really suggest that anyone with emetophobia talks to someone about it because there will be people out there who understand and have the same fear.'

Personally, I've always tended to hide behind humour. So, I would explain the impact my emetophobia had on me and then laugh and shrug it off. The trouble with that attitude is it means people don't take it seriously. If you go to your doctor and explain that emetophobia is ruining your life with a big grin and a chuckle, they're hardly likely to feel your need for support is desperate. You're probably more likely to be taken seriously if you burst into tears while talking about it. Not my style but a more effective way of communicating the severity of the problem and your need for help.

If you can be open about your anxiety, it will also give your friends and family a helpful insight into your behaviour. For example, if someone invites you out for dinner and you say no because you don't like eating in restaurants, it's much better if they understand that's the reason you turned them down. If they know about your emetophobia they are much more likely to say they would love to hang out and to ask what you would feel comfortable doing. Win-win situation.

Sharing your struggles with the right people can also make you feel much less alone and much better supported. Living with, and recovering from, emetophobia is not easy – don't choose to do it by yourself. You'll probably find those closest to you are touched that you trust them with your anxieties and are keen to help you in any way they can.

I didn't follow my own advice. When I was younger, I kept my emetophobia to myself, as much as was conceivably possible, and it was a bad idea. Only recently, in my thirties, and now that I am largely recovered, have I felt able to talk openly about it...and to write about it. I still find it tricky though – a large part of me wants to hide under the bed and never come out when I think about this book becoming public.

As I've said before, things were a bit different when I was a teenager, and people didn't talk about mental health nearly as openly as they do now. Nonetheless, it was a bad shout. Not that it was really a conscious decision. I was just like the people described above – I felt embarrassed and ashamed of admitting to it. I didn't know how to talk about it and didn't like to show any weakness.

Of course, it was obvious to my family and friends that I was struggling, that I wasn't eating properly and that I was losing weight, but I didn't talk about it and brushed off any questions. How much better it would have been if I'd felt able to tell them what was going on. All efforts my poor parents made to address the issue with me, I immediately dismissed, probably rudely. So how on earth were they supposed to know what was going on or what needed to be done? I also clearly remember shouting at a doctor to 'leave me alone' when she asked me one probing question too many.

While it may be hard, it's important to keep looking outwards. This helps you to remain connected and feel close to people, and allows those around you to help you challenge your emetophobic thoughts and behaviours. If you never speak about it or discuss it with anyone, it can snowball in your mind. You need the input of people without the condition to keep you grounded in 'normality' and aware of how other people perceive the risk of being sick. They can act as invaluable sense checkers. You know the deal – sitting stewing in your own thoughts doesn't tend to help. Much better to let the thoughts of others in.

* * *

Experts now understand that it's genuinely impossible for people with emetophobia to use logic and reason to reduce their anxiety. So, the more therapists, doctors, parents and friends try to insist on rationality, the more frustrated everyone will get, and it will be completely futile anyway.[4] This can be extremely challenging for anyone trying to help someone overcome their emetophobia and is another reason why open and honest communication is the best policy. The people around you need to understand that you aren't difficult, unreasonable or downright pig-headed – you genuinely can't help it and aren't doing it on purpose. But persuading someone who has never had the condition is no mean feat and can, sadly, lead to great conflict, particularly between parents and their emetophobic children.

This is a scene you may well be familiar with. It is, for example, typical for a family meal for many young people with emetophobia to go like this: parent spends ages lovingly cooking a delicious and nutritious meal that they believe their child will like, because they are desperate to look after and nourish them. Teen refuses to do more than pick at the potato/pasta/rice/insert-any-other-bland-and-low-risk carbohydrate. Well-meaning parent gets frustrated, upset, worried and, eventually, angry. Teen clams up, refuses to eat or engage in constructive conversation before storming off to their room feeling guilty for upsetting their parent, ashamed of their illness, angry with themselves, and a failure. Parent is left worried sick (excuse the pun) and throwing away the perfectly good food they had poured their heart into producing. Lose-lose situation. Upsetting for all parties but no one's fault.

The only solution is to be as open and honest with your friends and family as you can manage. They are much better able to support you, and to be understanding, if you explain to them how you are feeling and what you are struggling with. Opting for the stony silence route that I went for doesn't help anyone.

Even if you've explained clearly what you're going through, you may need to be patient with those around you to an extent. I'm sure they will do their best to support you, but the reality is that even for the most angelic character, it can be very frustrating supporting someone with a condition like this. I like to think that I'm well placed to support my children if they're feeling anxious because I get it. However, it troubles me that I have seen frustration in myself many times when, for example, one of them has been anxious and refused to eat any sensible food. However much you get it and want to be loving and supportive, it's extremely hard to stay calm, especially if you're already busy and stressed, and not say something along the lines of, 'Just eat your effing dinner!'

What would happen if I told my doctor about my symptoms?

There's something else I want to address here. I think one of the reasons I didn't talk about my emetophobia when I was a teenager was that I feared what would happen. I was scared that I'd be packed off to some kind of institution, or that I'd be force-fed medication and frog-marched to a shrink. It was about control – I didn't want to lose control of my life and my illness. As we know, people with emetophobia are generally not keen on the idea of losing control!

I spoke to NHS general practitioner (GP), Dr Guy Benison-Horner, to find out what would actually happen if you went to see your doctor about emetophobia. I asked him what an appointment with a patient with severe anxiety is generally like.

Dr Benison-Horner explained that you would probably be asked a range of questions about your symptoms and how they impact your life. He said by asking these questions the doctor aims to find out how severe the symptoms are as this will influence the treatment plan going forward. He explained that doctors will often go through anxiety questionnaires with you as these help assess the severity of your condition.

The doctor said on the NHS in the UK most people presenting with these symptoms will be referred, if they wish, for CBT, or other forms of therapy. If there's one available, they may also be offered appointments with a specialist mental health nurse. These sessions would give you the opportunity to talk through your anxieties and to discuss strategies for coping with them.

Dr Benison-Horner told me that medication may also be an option for some patients if their symptoms are debilitating. See Chapter 7 for more on treatment and medication.

The doctor reassured me that patients over the age of about twelve are generally considered to have the capacity to make decisions about their medical care and that, within reason, these decisions must be respected by their doctor. Neither medics nor parents have the right to overrule them. In other words, the chances are that you will have full control over what treatment you receive after careful discussion with your doctor.

Dr Benison-Horner also explained that the only time a patient might lose the right to make decisions about their own care is if they are deemed to be a serious risk to their own life, or to that of someone else.

Generally, he said, this would only apply in cases of psychosis (not relevant to emetophobia), extreme malnutrition (a BMI of less than 15 – usually only seen in anorexia) or an immediate risk of suicide.

To be clear, just telling your doctor that you have suicidal thoughts wouldn't result in anything more than an urgent referral to the mental health team. More drastic intervention would only be taken if the doctor thought you were going to harm yourself immediately on leaving the building.

Behaviours that might lead them to get this impression include having made clear plans to end your life, having written suicide notes, having said goodbye to people, or believing that you would be doing others a favour if you took your own life.

Finally, Dr Benison-Horner explained, 'A doctor at their best is trying to be open and to start a conversation about options – trying to ask questions that are open, non-intrusive and friendly, and which build trust.'

In other words, the doctor's job is to nurture a safe and informed dialogue in which you can describe how you are feeling and discuss the potential solutions, and which are best for you.

Dating and relationships

Okay, we've considered friends, and we've learned that you're perfectly safe being open about your anxiety, so let's now look at the impact of emetophobia on romantic relationships. My experience on this topic is, admittedly, limited. As I've said, I didn't have anything in the way of a love life before I went to university and there, I soon gained a boyfriend who is now my husband, so I'm no great authority on dating. However, I'm sorry to be boring but the same rule applies here as it did with friends – it's best to be open and honest with a partner, or potential partner, so they can understand you and your current situation.

I mean, I wouldn't necessarily open the conversation on a first date with, 'By the way, I have a debilitating fear of vom', but you're probably best off not trying to hide it for too long. After all, any serious partner is going to notice pretty fast, so you may as well be frank about it. Being able to talk about this kind of issue will lead to a much stronger and closer relationship with the right person anyway.

If they love you, or even just have a huge crush on you, and want to be with you, they will accept everything about you, and your emetophobia won't come between you. If they aren't willing to love you and support you through it, then they probably aren't the right person for you in the long run.

I'm trying to recall when, or how, I told Jamie about my emetophobia. I can't remember. I think it probably came out gradually. I don't think we had any sort of big reveal moment. He must have noticed little signs of it over time. I certainly didn't try to hide it from him and I'm glad about that – I think I was just, well, me. It's never really been an issue in our relationship, except, maybe, for the odd moment when my controlling behaviour around food has frustrated him. I suspect, also, that he'd pick more exotic holiday destinations if left to his own devices!

Zoe explained that when she was first dating her husband, he spent ages cooking her a special dinner but that he cooked carbonara with raw egg, so she felt unable to eat it. She said, 'I felt so bad because he was hurt and upset. It has a huge impact on the other person in a relationship.'

Zoe added that it upsets her that she now sometimes sees her husband adopting some of her anxieties. For example, she said he was eating prawns, and she could see him examining them in the way she would.

She said, 'I really don't like how he's now seeing things that I see – threats that aren't really there.'

But, to take a step backwards from marriage for a moment, how does emetophobia impact flirting and the initial stages of a new partnership? Obviously, all relationships are different, and they start in various ways. It seems to me, though, that flirting with someone involves an element of relaxed playfulness and that's a vibe hard to achieve while feeling very anxious.

When my emetophobia was severe, and I was debilitatingly anxious, I think I unintentionally built a wall around myself. It was a kind of self-protective, controlling barrier behind which I hid. I still do sometimes. I imagine it made me come across as cold and distant. That state is the opposite to a flirtatious one. If all your energy is being absorbed by anxiety, and a bid to maintain control, it's impossible to let go and be free and joyful enough to engage in flirtation.

Try to be gentle with yourself about this – don't beat yourself up if you're finding it hard. You're on a journey (cliché alert!) and what is difficult now won't necessarily always be. And, anyway, beautiful relationships can develop without any playful flirtation. All you can do is be the best version of your current self and keep working on recovery... See Chapter 7.

Intimacy

Say you find a partner; this is where the next challenge can arise. It's common for people with emetophobia to struggle with intimacy because they fear they will be sick midway through, or because they worry their partner may be ill and that by kissing them, they will catch a virus.

Time for me to repeat myself again – talk to them. If you avoid kissing your partner, they are likely to think you aren't attracted to them, or that they have bad breath or something. Tell them the truth so they know it isn't personal and that it doesn't mean you don't fancy them. Discuss it and try to find a solution, or compromise, that works for both of you.

Consensual sex is, of course, often a very important part of a relationship for those who are old enough, but there are plenty of other forms of closeness that can be equally intimate, but which may feel less threatening. For example, holding hands, cuddling while watching TV or giving each other a massage can all help with bonding and attachment and give both parties a welcome hit of the 'cuddle chemical' oxytocin.[5]

Pregnancy

You might well feel a million miles away from this being relevant, but the other thing we should mention, for if and when it becomes relevant, is babies. It's well recognised that some people with emetophobia want to have children but avoid pregnancy for fear of morning sickness. For those who find this to be a concern, clear communication with a partner is again vital so that they understand your worries. If you think you might want to get pregnant later in your life but are worried about morning sickness, many find this to be a powerful motivator for tackling emetophobia. See Chapter 7 for more information on treatment and overcoming emetophobia.

Fun

So that's friendships and dating. What about social lives? Emetophobia has a charming way of making anything that should be fun, not fun. Even the most amazing party in the world isn't fun if you feel very sick, are constantly on the verge of a panic attack and can think about nothing other than whether you are going to throw up.

Obviously, how badly your social life is affected depends on how severe your emetophobia is and which symptoms are particularly problematic for you. Let's be honest, fun and full-blown emetophobia are probably mutually exclusive. So, let's accept that while working towards recovery, and let's focus on small wins.

Partying or a sleepover with your mates may not be possible yet. Emphasis on yet! But what is possible? Where can little hits of fun be found? Try not to berate yourself for struggling with big, or impressive, TikTok-worthy social blowouts. Right now, any fun or enjoyment that can be found is well worth having. Just a few minutes spent doing something you are actively enjoying can brighten your whole day and improve your frame of mind. For example, for me, running through the countryside in the sun puts a huge grin on my face and allows me to briefly forget everything else. Even just ten minutes can completely transform my mood.

Now, I'm quite prepared to accept that running isn't everyone's idea of fun, but could you try setting aside half an hour, or an hour, a day to do something you can enjoy, or have fun doing, despite your anxiety? It doesn't matter what it is – anything you enjoy is great. Maybe watching a comedy sketch online, chatting to a friend on the phone, or playing a ball game in the garden or park. Whatever floats your boat.

There will be plenty of time for the pyjama parties, sports trips and living it up once you're feeling better. At this point, you could just make a list of all the things you would like to do once your emetophobia is under control. This sort of bucket list can act as a powerful motivator to help you stick with treatment – it's something to aim for.

My top tips for socialising with emetophobia

Now, without further ado, here are my top tips for keeping your social life afloat until you have escaped your emetophobia:

- Be honest and open. You (obviously) don't need to tell everyone your whole life story and every thought but tell a few close friends and/or family as much as you feel comfortable sharing. It prevents incorrect, and potentially damaging, assumptions being made and allows them to support you.

- Be realistic about what social events you can manage and enjoy. If someone invites you to meet for lunch and you know you will struggle with the food, say you would love to see them but ask if coffee would work instead of lunch. Or a drink in a cafe instead of dinner. Maybe a walk instead of a cinema trip? Whatever makes you most comfortable. In other words, don't give an outright 'no', because you don't want people to get the impression you don't want to spend time with them (unless, that is, you really don't want to see that particular person) – just adjust plans to give you the best chance of enjoying yourself.

- Consider joining a club, or sports team, or taking up a hobby, that would get you out and about regularly to spend time doing something you enjoy with friends, or people who could become friends. An ideal activity is one where you commit to being part of a team that you don't want to let down. If you're anything like me, this would make you less likely to bail on the back of an anxious thought.

- Look for little wins. They may seem insignificant, but they add up and make a big difference. Twenty minutes laughing and playing with a goofy dog in the sunshine may not be your idea of a spectacular adventure, but if it makes you smile, it's enough to raise your spirits and give you a boost.

- Challenge yourself. Push yourself just enough to keep your options as wide open as possible, but without triggering panic attacks and misery. The more you allow the emetophobic voice in your head to call the shots, the smaller your world will become. So, you need to push back as much as you can – but without completely freaking yourself out. So, for example, if someone proposes a trip and your immediate reaction is, 'Help, panic, no can do, how do I get out of it?' maybe pause for a moment and ask yourself whether you can override that voice and do it anyway. If you really can't, then by all means say no for now, but just take a moment to consider it first.

Conclusion

So, that's the deal with navigating relationships, social life and communication when you have emetophobia. Next, we will consider the challenges of school and work. After all, attending school when you have debilitating anxiety is something of an expert subject of mine, as you will see.

Chapter 5

SURVIVING SCHOOL AND WORK

We've now looked at how emetophobia can impact your relationship with food, your friendships and your love life. As we continue our exploration of life with this condition, it's time to consider your education and career.

How does emetophobia impact education and careers?

Emetophobia can cause a range of difficulties in both school and work life. But what are those difficulties? How does this condition impact students and employees? Indeed, how is it impacting your work or study?

Time for some bullet points, I'd say...

- Emetophobia can make you so anxious you can't focus on your work.
- It can make you feel too afraid to attend work or school at all, or to go on away days, school trips or business trips.

- It can cause disordered eating, which can be problematic in the school canteen, at business lunches, at networking breakfasts and the like.
- It can cause panic attacks, which may strike at unhelpful moments, such as while you're trying to give a presentation or when you're asking your boss for a pay rise.
- It can make you want to run screaming from a meeting or lesson if someone says they aren't feeling well.
- The phobia can cause avoidance and safety-seeking behaviours, which may be noticed by colleagues or classmates. For example, it might draw comment if you wash your hands multiple times a day, or if you avoid lecture theatres even when there's an important talk taking place.

These are just some examples of how emetophobia can impact people. There are many other ways in which emetophobia can affect people in their education and careers. Maybe you can think of other impacts it's having on you?

Zoe said she would have loved to be a doctor but that her emetophobia completely ruled that option out because medics are inevitably exposed to people who are unwell and who might vomit.

She explained, 'It definitely impacted my career choice. I'm a lawyer – law was a safe bet. It's sad to admit, really.'

Zoe is unusual in that she's open about her emetophobia at work. She said that all her colleagues are aware of it and she has made it a rule within her team that if anyone is sick, they work from home for three days. She added laughingly that her colleagues think this is great.

She said, 'Work are respectful of it. They're great. They know it's not a joke. In fact, I'm not in the office today because one of my colleagues was sick at the weekend. If I went in, I would be trying to keep my distance – it takes a lot of mental energy so it's easier to work from home.'

As for me, my emetophobia developed when I was at school. I will explain...

My experience of emetophobia at school

From the age of fourteen onwards my emetophobia got progressively worse. Gradually, I became more and more unwell. By the time I was in the last year of school, I could barely sleep or eat, I was having constant panic attacks, had chronic, overwhelming nausea and was significantly underweight.

Each morning, I'd retch and shake violently the whole way to school, and I couldn't concentrate on my lessons because I felt so sick. I could hardly drive I was so panicked – I certainly shouldn't have been driving – and the writing in my school folders was illegible because my hand was always shaking so hard.

All my energy and focus were constantly on my internal panic, trying to avoid throwing up, and looking for the best possible escape routes to use if I were to be sick. It's impossible to focus on the minutiae of glacial landforms, while wondering at exactly which moment one will need to leg it from the room to throw up.

Every day I desperately wanted to find any excuse not to go to school. The emetophobic voice in my head would SCREAM at me constantly not to risk it. Not to go. It was like trying to force myself to walk naked into a den of starving lions. Every ounce of willpower I could muster was required just to make myself drive to school each morning. Literally anything seemed preferable to going to school. Because going to school meant risking being sick at school, and that was the worst thing imaginable.

So desperate was I to get out of the cycle of anxious school days, of repeated jumps from the metaphorical plane, I even tried to lose enough weight that I'd be hospitalised, as sitting in hospital seemed a better option. To be honest, I didn't have to try very hard – as I was too anxious to eat the weight was falling off anyway.

It was only my absolute determination to do well in my exams, and to have a shot at Oxford or Cambridge University, that kept me dragging myself in every day.

By this time, I was so anxious about the risk of food poisoning, and viewed all food as so hazardous, that my diet dwindled to a nutritious (!) combination of white bread, Jaffa Cakes and the occasional cereal bar.

I was also increasingly self-destructive and suicidal, self-harming and getting some sort of twisted pleasure from seeing the weight fall off. Not because I thought I was overweight but, I think, because I needed a visible manifestation of my internal suffering. Or maybe just because I wanted to destroy myself in whatever way I could. It was the only way out I could see from the torment my emetophobia was causing me. Yes, that was what it boiled down to. Destroying myself was the only conceivable way to escape the daily torture of living with the emetophobia.

But how on earth did I get into that state?

When I was in the penultimate year, I loved school. Yes, I did feel anxious and nauseous, but it wasn't all-consuming. I expected my time in the final year to be the same. I knew I'd have to contend with anxiety, knew it was part of my life at that time, but assumed it would be like what I'd experienced and managed before.

Then something changed. It was the end of the summer holidays between the last two years of school, and I'd missed school during the break. Dare I say it, I was also quite looking forward to getting stuck into my exam courses. But as August drew to a close, I realised I wasn't looking forward to the new school year. Actually, I was dreading it, and I didn't understand why. Something had shifted within me. It was as though a dark, insidious ghost had wormed its way inside me and quietly staged a coup.

We were on holiday in Cornwall when this realisation began to dawn on me. The weather was perfect and we were staying in a charming, family hotel overlooking the sea with fabulous beaches and endless opportunities for walking, swimming, cycling, paddleboarding and sunbathing, but I was repeatedly confined to my hotel room by crippling panic attacks. I was desperate not to get to the end of the holiday. Not to have to go home. Because going home meant going back to school.

Day after day on that trip my parents tried to persuade me to go out walking, cycling or exploring with them and my brothers. But I couldn't. I wanted to. I would have. But every time I contemplated going, the anxious voice in my head would scream at me and I'd have to say no.

What if you are sick when you are out?

What if you get an upset stomach and aren't near a loo?

Better to stay safely in the hotel room near the bathroom.

Anything that happens can't be embarrassing if you are in the hotel by yourself.

Safer to be alone than in company.

My family must have thought I was being a typically grumpy, difficult teenager on that holiday. But there, in my nautical-themed hotel room, my heart would be pounding, stomach churning, mind whirring. I'd pace up and down past the bed with its blue and white duvet and matching scatter cushions desperately trying to regain control of myself. I'd try reading, or watching TV, but wouldn't be able to concentrate or sit still. I'd have to get up and keep moving. Keep breathing. Remind myself it would pass. Just hang on in there...

Basically, I wasn't at all well, was I? I wasn't well enough for the pressure of exams and university application. But I didn't know that, and nor did anyone else. That malignant ghost was now the dictator of my body. I didn't exist any longer. I had left nothing behind but an empty shell of a body which kind of looked a bit like me but was ruled by another power entirely.

But, anyway, to get back to the point, what I was trying to say was that as I returned to school for my final year, the pressure was on, and I wasn't up to handling it.

What help did I need?

I have been asked many times, and, indeed, have asked myself many times, what I needed when I was at school. What would have helped me? Until recently I've found myself unable to answer that question.

I needed therapy but I wasn't ready to receive it. I didn't want it so it wouldn't have helped. Why didn't I want it? Well, because my emetophobia was my safety net and so, much as it was tormenting me, I don't think I wanted to lose it. It was protecting me from the thing I feared most.

Also, I was very self-destructive – I didn't want to get better. If anything, I wanted to get worse. Why? I don't know. Maybe that was a symptom of the illness? But the thing is, the result was that however much I objectively needed therapy, I didn't want to receive it. Or wasn't well enough to do so.

People have also asked what my school could have done to help me. Yes, they turned a blind eye to me skipping assembly and they let me sit my exams in a room by myself, so I didn't have to face the big exam hall. Was that the right thing for them to do? If you ask a therapist, then maybe not. Because if you avoid situations which make you anxious, the fear perpetuates, and you never learn that those settings are safe.

Thing is, though, it's all academic really, because I was ill and I needed serious medical treatment – the odd bit of assembly skipping was neither here nor there. I wasn't trying to tackle my emetophobia – I was just trying to survive each day.

The other factor at play here was that I was in my final year of school and taking my exams. That was important. I believed there was no way I could have focused on getting my grades and on tackling my emetophobia in the same year. That would have been far too much to ask of anyone, let alone of anyone already unwell. Therefore, I have to conclude that the best thing for me that year was just to be nursed through until I had my exams done and was free to concentrate on my recovery.

But what I'm coming to is that I think there was only one thing that might have helped when I was finishing school; in fact, it was the intervention that did eventually turn things around, that finally got me ready to receive proper treatment and to start getting better. That, for me, was medication. The chemical shift antidepressants caused within me improved my mental health sufficiently that I was able to engage with treatment and that I started to want to get better. Without them, it was hopeless for me. You're never going to get better if you don't want to.

We'll explore this properly later in the book but there was a catch 22. I believe the only thing that would have helped me in my final years of school was medication. However, my GP wouldn't give that to me until I was older. As Dr Guy Benison-Horner told me, doctors are very reluctant to prescribe antidepressants to teenagers because of the potential side effects. If that's the case now, it was even more so when I was at school.

So, while it was awful, maybe the way things played out was the best way they could have done. I survived to the end of school, I took my exams, and I received the medication I needed from my doctor as soon as I was old enough. It's comforting to conclude that it probably worked out as well as it could have.

However, had I been under the care of a psychiatrist, rather than just a primary care doctor, I may have been prescribed the meds sooner. If you think you need medication to enable you to take part in emetophobia treatment, it is definitely worth consulting a psychiatrist as they may prescribe them when primary care doctors won't.

Work

While my emetophobia primarily impacted my time at school, plenty of people struggle with it at work, be that in their career or in part-time or holiday jobs. You may have questions about how to handle your emetophobia at work. I'll do my best to answer some of the more commonly asked questions:

Should I tell my boss about my emetophobia?

The answer depends on how much of an impact the condition is having on your work life. If it isn't having much bearing, there's no need to mention it. If, however, it is making you very anxious at work, or if it's causing you to struggle in certain situations at work, then it is definitely worth mentioning it and asking whether it's possible to discuss ways in which you might be able to amend your work commitments to make your life easier.

How should I tell my boss?

This depends a bit on what sort of job you have and what the setup is like. Generally, though, it's best to make an appointment with your boss for a time that suits them, when you can discuss it in private and neither of you is in a hurry or likely to be interrupted. It's then best to explain briefly what emetophobia is, how it's impacting you at work and how your boss can help. You might also consider printing out some information about the condition to give them so they can learn more about the phobia, as the chances are they'll never have heard of it.

What about my colleagues?

This really comes down to how private a person you are, the social dynamic in your workplace and how close you are to your colleagues. There is no need to tell your colleagues about your emetophobia unless it is having a direct impact on the way you work, or interact, with them. Indeed, personally, I think I would rather my colleagues' view of me was based on the quality of my work and how I am to work with, rather than on my mental health, but that's just me. So, sure, if you've got close friends at work and want to talk to them about it, then go for it. If not, that's fine too.

Managing anxiety at school and work

Concentrating on school or your work is impossible when you're feeling very anxious or panicky. You haven't a hope of focusing on anything other than your internal turmoil. So, how can you reduce your anxiety levels in the moment, while at work, school, college or university?

Well, you could, of course, try stepping outside for a few moments of fresh air – to 'take a breather'. Or you could pause what you're doing and spend five minutes 'breaking state' and going to get a glass of water that you could sip quietly.

There are plenty of other scientifically proven options you could also try out. Most involve breathing and are easy to do quickly in an office or classroom without anyone around you noticing. Why don't you give some of these tried and tested strategies a go and see what helps you?

- 3-4-5 breathing – Dr Chatterjee recommends breathing exercises as a way of almost immediately flipping you from fight or flight mode into a state of comparative relaxation. This technique simply involves breathing in for three seconds, holding your breath for four seconds and then breathing out for five seconds.[1]
- Box breathing – Like 3-4-5 breathing, this technique can help lower your stress levels and calm your nervous

system. All you have to do is to breathe in for four seconds, then hold your breath for four, and then breathe out for four seconds.[2]

- Deep breathing – The simplest of all the options, just focus on breathing in and out slowly and deeply for a few minutes.

- The 3-3-3 rule – This technique involves employing a range of different senses to reduce your anxiety by distracting your attention. First, look around you and name three things you can see, then listen to the sounds around you and name three things you can hear. Finally, move three parts of your body.

- Count backwards – Sit quietly, maybe close your eyes, and count slowly backwards from a hundred to zero.

- Exercise – Go for a short, brisk walk, preferably outside. Being in nature is calming and exercise helps discharge tension and reduce stress and anxiety.

Stigma

I didn't receive any formal support or help when I was at school, but I was treated kindly insomuch as I was treated at all. Sadly, this isn't always the case. So, before we look at how to keep your education or career on track while living with emetophobia, I think we need to address the issue of mental health stigma.

Thankfully, with every passing year this is becoming less of a problem. It's much less prevalent now than when I was a teenager and will be even less so in five years' time. That's great. I get, though, that it does still exist.

Especially with little-known conditions like emetophobia, it can be hard to get people to take you seriously, or to get them to understand how debilitating it is. If someone has Alzheimer's no explanation is needed, but there isn't always the same understanding of mental health conditions like emetophobia.

The best way to break down stigma is through sharing information. So, if you experience stigma, misunderstanding or people not being empathetic, the best thing to do is to educate them, if you feel able to do this. Explain what it means to live with emetophobia and share information from reputable sources[3] such as the EmetAction or Anxiety UK websites in the UK, or the Anxiety and Depression Association of America. In doing so, you will help to end the remaining stigmas and make the world a better place for everyone.

Ellie's emetophobia was so severe that she missed weeks of school. She said, 'I felt trapped in every situation, I wouldn't let anyone near me, I was scared of touching anything, I didn't want to leave the house, and I couldn't go to school. I didn't go in for quite a few weeks, but no one understood how scared I was. In the end, my mum went into school and explained what was going on and what they needed to do. I just had to lay it out clearly – to communicate it – and then they were supportive and understanding.'

In other words, explaining clearly what she was going through ensured Ellie didn't experience stigma and was well supported when she returned to school.

Experiencing stigma, or negative reactions from friends and family – you know, the 'pull yourself together and stop complaining' mindset – can be very upsetting and disempowering. In fact, it can be downright devastating. A thick skin is required for coping with people dismissing, or even mocking, something that is tormenting you.

Aside from educating and explaining, there isn't a huge amount you can do about the reactions of people you know. But what do you do if you experience stigma at school, college or work? Especially if it's impacting your education or career, it's crucial to nip it in the bud as soon as possible.

Under the UK's Equality Act of 2010, it's illegal to discriminate against people with a disability.[4] Other countries have similar legislation – it's worth looking up what rules apply where you live. You may well not view your emetophobia as a disability, I certainly don't, but under this legislation a mental health condition counts as a disability if it has a significant impact on your ability to carry out day-to-day activities.[5]

This means it's illegal, say, for your employer not to give you a promotion purely because of your emetophobia or the behaviours it causes. Or it would apply if you were teased about your safety-seeking behaviours at school or work. Basically, any situation in which you are upset, or held back by, people's reaction to your emetophobia could be illegal under this Act and should be addressed.

Here is a simple example: you apply for a job and are up against another candidate with the same skills, grades and qualifications but the other applicant is given the job simply because you declare on the application form that you have an anxiety disorder.

Assuming that was the only reason they were given the job instead of you, that's illegal under the Equality Act. If, of course, you not only declare you have anxiety disorder but that you also have an addiction to shoplifting, enjoy slaughtering baby animals and make a habit of starting fires in national parks, that might be a different matter...

The Act also means that if you inform your employer of your 'disability' they are required to take appropriate measures to ensure you can do the job despite it. For example, if you tell them about your emetophobia, they may have to let you skip work events that involve international travel.

If you experience discrimination, you have a range of options. The first and least involved is simply to raise your concern with your school or employer informally.[6] Often this is enough to resolve the issue, especially given you have the law on your side, and few organisations relish the idea of a lawsuit against them.

However, if the problem persists, you can make a formal complaint using your organisation's complaints procedure or you can even take legal action.[7]

* * *

As we have now seen, emetophobia and the stigma around it can have a profound impact on a person's education and career. It's crucial to be aware of the impact it's having on you, and to take steps to minimise the effect, because, as Dr Alexandra Keyes and Professor David Veale say, 'If your emetophobia is very severe and you miss out on many things in life such as relationships, education, career and social life, you may have developed a depression which is secondary to your emetophobia.'[8]

In other words, if your emetophobia is holding you back in life, due to stigma or not, that can have a knock-on effect on other aspects of your wellbeing and quality of life, so it needs to be addressed. See Chapter 7!

Zara said that she did a work experience placement in a primary school and found it really difficult when norovirus went around the nursery. She said she was sanitising and washing her hands all the time in a bid to protect herself. She's now doing a placement as a student physio in a hospital and she raised her emetophobia with her tutors and they were unaware of it. However, happily, she didn't feel stigmatised. She said her tutors reassured her that they had very rarely seen anyone be sick while they were working in hospitals.

Nonetheless, Zara said she feels panicked if she is going to see a patient whose notes mention they've vomited or if they tell her they are feeling nauseous. However, she added, 'I have to plough on because you can't deny someone care because they're sick – but not overthinking is hard.'

Remy added that she works in a bar and that if anyone is sick, she has to run outside to avoid being sick herself. She said there is no way she could tidy up after a drunk customer is sick; hearing someone being sick can make her vomit, and that in turn makes her cry. She said the only solution is to hide outside when that happens.

What if I'm not in work or education?

Before we wrap this chapter up, there's something important to say: in this section so far, I've only focused on people who are in either education, training or employment. Of course, that, quite wrongly, leaves a lot of people out. Maybe you're unemployed or taking a gap year or choosing not to work. Or, maybe, you're desperate to be in school or work but can't be currently because of the severity of your emetophobia.

If this applies to you, the first and most important thing you can do is to try to tackle your emetophobia – to recover sufficiently that you are able to return to work or education. See Chapter 7 for how to do this.

You will, I imagine, need time to work with a therapist on overcoming the condition and you may, also, need to experiment with medication. This is an excellent time to learn more about how to look after yourself as well as possible to improve your general wellbeing, as this can only help in your recovery. See Chapter 8 for more on self-care.

Once you feel able, I would suggest looking for a role that seems as manageable as possible – take things a step at a time. Challenge yourself but set challenges that are achievable. As you get better, you can up the difficulty of the challenge. So, maybe, you might initially look for a job that allows you to work from home. Then you might move to a part-time role based somewhere near your house.

I hope the tips in this chapter will be useful to you if you do eventually decide to return to education or employment; if not, you can always rip these pages out and use them as firelighters or wrapping paper.

But the point is, if you aren't working because of your emetophobia, but wish that you were, skip to Chapter 7 for information on how to recover from this condition. Then you can always return to this chapter as and when it's relevant.

Even if you're currently missing out on the education or career opportunities you'd like, don't worry – you'll be able to catch up once you are well enough. Your wellbeing is always the most important thing. The rest can be sorted out one way or another. And, from what I've observed, your experience with this condition will leave you a more empathetic, deep and wise person who will be a pleasure to work with in the future.

My top tips for surviving school and work with emetophobia

Finally, if you are in education or employment, what can you do to thrive until you have recovered from your emetophobia?

Here are my suggestions:

- If you experience any form of stigma or discrimination at work or school, be brave and tackle it ASAP. Don't go straight in all guns blazing – try to resolve it peacefully – but use all available channels to ensure that you are being treated fairly.

- Do as much as you can as 'normally' as you can but be open about anything you're finding difficult and discuss tweaks to help you cope. For me, this was being allowed to miss assembly and taking exams in a separate room rather than in the main exam hall. These things certainly didn't make my life easy, but they took the pressure off a tiny bit.

- Don't expect, or demand, too much of yourself – if you have a huge project on or are sitting exams, it probably isn't the right moment to take on your emetophobia. Wait until things are quieter at work, school or university so you have the headspace to address the phobia properly.

- Confide in a trustworthy colleague, teacher or schoolmate. Explain to them what you are going through. This will give you an ally. Even just an understanding smile from them when you are struggling will help.

- Make your employer aware of your emetophobia so they take it into account and accommodate for it.

- Remember to frame things positively – yes you might

be highly strung and need a bit of leeway, but this trait means you probably have other positive characteristics as an employee.

So, that's how emetophobia can impact your eating habits, social life, education and career. We now need to go on a little diversion to look at how to stay safe online while living with, and recovering from, the condition.

Chapter 6

PROTECTING YOURSELF IN THE DIGITAL WORLD

Misinformation

I just spent five minutes scrolling through my Instagram feed. I learned that camels' humps are full of raisins, Princess Diana is spending the weekend with her grandchildren, and Donald Trump has grown a new ear. Where do I start? Maybe with the fact Princess Diana died nearly thirty years ago? None of these things are true.

This is a trap it's important to be aware of when reading about emetophobia online. If you went back twenty years to when I developed emetophobia, you would find virtually nothing on the internet about the condition. Indeed, nor would you find any books about it in the library. Thankfully, there's a lot of helpful, and accurate, information available these days, which is fabulous. There's also a lot of nonsense.

It's a bit of a jungle out there so you need to be clued up in order to protect yourself from going down unhelpful rabbit holes. Your best bet is to stick to reading, and watching, content from reliable sources, such as the NHS website in the UK, the websites of mental health charities, and of well-regarded treatment centres. See the Further Reading section for more ideas.

As for social media content, be aware that much of it is produced by people with no legitimate qualifications. These people may be absolutely correct in what they are sharing, but it's hard to be sure. The best bet is to stick to advice and information provided by charities and therapists – this is the most reliable. The further off the beaten track you go, the greater your risk of running into rubbish. And, let's be honest, when you're grappling with this beast, the last thing you need is bad advice or inaccurate information.

Something you should be particularly wary of on social media is people claiming to have...or more likely be selling...quick-fix, simple cures for emetophobia. Sadly, the reality is that there's no such thing as a magic bullet cure for this condition. As we will see in the next chapter, the only option is CBT with exposure therapy, possibly in conjunction with medication. Anyone claiming to have any better options should be treated with extreme caution. If it sounds too good to be true, it probably is.

For example, I found someone claiming to be able to cure emetophobia with eight weeks of treatment. I haven't tried their treatment so I can't know for sure that this is misleading. However, the experts generally reckon it takes a couple of years to recover, so...

Social media

In the last chapter we looked at the importance of close friends and relationships. Social media complicates this a little. Increasingly, people are spending their time interacting on social media instead of in person. This may well be more comfortable for you if your emetophobia is making you very anxious – you can chat to people on Snapchat from the comfort of your own home.

However, interactions on social media are no substitute for seeing real people, in person, giving them a hug and having a deep and meaningful chat.[1] This is partly because, without the checks of body language and facial expression, people often say things in digital messages that they wouldn't dream of saying in person. You know, snide remarks, insulting comments, that sort of thing. The problem with this is it's a source of stress, leaves a feeling of hurt and rejection and can lower mood and increase anxiety.[2] Put simply, if you're already struggling, having someone criticise your online post, whether it's about emetophobia or anything else, isn't going to improve your state of mind, is it?

Even if no one is unpleasant, posting something which doesn't gain many likes or comments can leave you feeling disappointed, unpopular or inadequate. This is a new form of social stress and one that can trigger a negative emotional reaction which you just don't need.[3] You know the feeling – when you check your phone and have no messages. It's often only a momentary sense of disappointment but that's enough to switch your brain into a stress state and to impact your wellbeing.

Basically, while it's fab if you have some fun interacting with nice, like-minded people on social media every now and then, if you can, it's better to hang out in person. After all, people were designed to live in closeknit tribes working together, supporting each other and being dependent on each other. The further we move from that way of life, the more stress is put on our minds, which simply can't keep up with the pace of change in modern life. Conversing on social media is fine, but not if it replaces time spent with friends in person.

Algorithms

In Chapter 3, we looked at how food rules tend to develop in people with emetophobia. We established that they're often triggered by information people have come across, such as reels about foods most likely to cause food poisoning. Okay. Keep that in mind. Now think about algorithms. People with emetophobia are more likely to click on articles, or posts, about illness, food hygiene, avoiding getting sick and so forth. Algorithms learn this. They then act on it. So, if you read a few of those stories, you will then be fed more and more of them. Soon your whole feed will be filled with stories about food poisoning outbreaks. This is neither helpful nor healthy. In fact, it's just downright misleading. It can skew your sense of how common, and how problematic, illness outbreaks are, which runs the risk of increasing your fear and desire for control.

Jamie is afraid of flying. As a result, he used to read all the articles about plane crashes, air safety, the mechanics of how planes stay in the sky and so on. So, if I looked at his social media feeds, I would find endless pictures of planes exploding in fireballs, crash landings and the like. If I then looked at my own social media, there wouldn't be a single mention of air travel, let alone of crashes. So, while Jamie was constantly being fed the message that flying is dangerous, I wasn't getting a hint of that. You see? It's the same for emetophobia.

So, outfox those sneaky algorithms – click on pictures of cute puppies, spectacular goals being scored by your favourite team, and delicious-looking recipes. Scroll straight past any triggering posts without a moment's pause. This is important because social media platforms measure the amount of time you spend looking at any given post to judge the extent of a response from you. They then use this data to determine which posts to show you – they want to feed you content that you will engage with. Be careful of these traps and then every time you pick up your phone you will be safe from further emetophobia-fuelling information.

Similarly, be aware that your online searches can add to the data companies hold on you and this can subsequently influence the content and adverts that you're shown. It's like the rumour that online supermarkets can tell if their customers are expecting a baby before the customers themselves know, purely based on their shopping habits.

The media

It's not only algorithms you need to watch out for. Anything that triggers a strong disgust response in people tends to get media, and social media, attention because it's useful clickbait. So, even if you aren't actively seeking these kinds of articles and content, editors probably are – they know they sell newspapers and encourage social media engagement. An obvious example is the number of articles published about norovirus outbreaks on cruise ships. We've all seen these stories, right? Well, how many stories have you seen about a cruise on which everything went smoothly, and no one got ill? None, of course. Because that's boring. It's not a story and it doesn't trigger a reaction in the reader. Engaging stories that get a response are what content producers are looking for. But it's deceptive. It gives the impression that a large proportion of cruises are impacted by vomiting outbreaks. That simply isn't true. So don't be put off cruises by a few articles.

I used to be a journalist, and my editor was keen on saying that every story we wrote should cause the reader to feel either angry, jealous or scared. I don't recollect ever being asked to write an article that would leave the reader feeling positive, good about the state of the world and filled with a sense of deep wellbeing.

The point is that editors and content creators aren't usually looking to give a completely balanced sense of what's going on in the world. If they were, their content would be extremely dull. They're looking to get clicks and sales. It's worth remembering that when you're on social media or looking at the news. The trouble is that even if you know that logically, these stories can still worm their way into your subconscious and make you anxious. What this means is that you'd probably be wise to think carefully about what content you expose yourself to. For me, I know that reading the news before bed is a bad idea. I want to be well informed about what's going on in the world, but I don't need scary intel ploughed into my brain just before sleep.

Forums and groups

Living with emetophobia can be lonely, especially if you're surrounded by people who don't seem to understand what you're going through. So, surely, being part of a community of people with the condition would be reassuring, supportive and helpful?

Well, possibly...but probably not.

There are lots of well-meaning people on emetophobia forums who respond to comments with empathy and the best tips they are aware of. So, sure, chatting to those people has its benefits – they can make you feel like you're not alone, that others understand your anxieties and that help is available. They may also offer genuinely useful suggestions and ideas based on their personal experience.

I've seen lots of comments by people offering concern, reassurance and support. Posts by people checking on how others are doing and encouraging them to seek the professional help they need. I've also seen messages with kind and positive thoughts about how achievable recovery from emetophobia is. So, forums certainly have their upsides.

However, unfortunately, there are a lot of downsides to forums which, I would argue, outweigh the benefits. First, they are hotbeds of panic. I've just been scrolling through some of the first sites that came up when I googled 'emetophobia forums'. I was hit by a barrage of terror and panic. Endless comments by people whose housemates were unwell, who had eaten something past its use by date or who felt ill. All these messages were by people with emetophobia in a state of panic. They were looking for reassurance. Okay, so you could login and offer some words of support or comfort. Sure. And that might make you feel good about yourself, momentarily, that you were able to help. But is it beneficial to you to be subjected to wave after wave of other people's anxiety? Not in my opinion.

Scrolling through these feeds brings thoughts of illness to the forefront of your mind, normalises the idea that vomiting is something to fear, and reinforces emetophobic thinking. For someone with emetophobia, seeing other people panic about vomit sends a message to the brain that it is, indeed, something to be afraid of. It would be much healthier, I think, to surround yourself with people who are totally chilled about it. The sort of people who shrug their shoulders and say, 'Oh well, I probably won't catch it and if I do, well, I'll live!' Those are the people who can help to subconsciously re-educate you and teach you a healthier reaction to the thought of illness.

Like social media, forums can be a bit of a black hole. Once you start scrolling through them, it's easy to get sucked in and to end up spending ages reading more and more posts. How are you going to feel after doing that? Full of the joys of spring? I don't think so. They're going to make you feel anxious and triggered. Reading other people's tales of woe may also make you feel depressed and hopeless. It isn't helpful to you to read all the anxieties other people have, how their lives have been ruined by emetophobia, or how every treatment they've tried has failed. I say, stick to your own path and keep working towards your own recovery. Don't allow other people to knock you off course.

Just as reading news articles or watching videos about norovirus outbreaks and the like can trigger the development of further avoidance behaviours and anxieties in people with emetophobia, forums can be a source of further rules. I just saw a post about the incubation period of various illnesses. Did reading that help me? No, it absolutely didn't. By reading it, all I've achieved is making myself worry that, maybe, I should feel anxious for even longer after being exposed to the risk of vomiting. Would I have been better off sticking to the forum discussing the best food for my dog? Yes, I would. Boring, but not damaging.

Finally, forums are almost exclusively full of other people with emetophobia who are, of course, experts by experience, but they aren't experts in the sense of people who are qualified and trained in the field. Many of them are very well informed and have a lot of experience of managing their emetophobia. However, they aren't necessarily a reliable source of information. Much better to stick to the advice of real experts, such as Dr Alexandra Keyes, Professor David Veale, Anna Christie and Dr David Russ, all of whom are psychologists, psychiatrists or counsellors with extensive experience of treating and researching emetophobia. These are the people whose expertise I have drawn on in researching and writing this book.

Artificial intelligence (AI)

Now, this is a whole new area but one which could become much bigger very quickly: AI therapy – essentially the use of chatbots to provide mental health support, often through specialist apps. These chatbots can use the principles of CBT to offer coping strategies and guidance to users. They can also help people identify negative thought patterns and can suggest ways to break those patterns. So far so good.

There are some notable benefits to AI therapy. For a start, no waiting lists, 24/7 availability, remote access and massively lower costs. Anyone who is struggling to afford, or access, therapy can get help immediately from a chatbot. Some people also find it easier to be open and honest with a chatbot than with a person, as they don't feel judged or scrutinised.

However, currently at least, despite the advantages, AI therapists are no substitute for human therapists. They can't offer real human empathy or connection, they have none of the years of training human therapists have, and they are not thought to be suitable for people with severe mental health conditions. It's also not recommended that they should be used without oversight from a real therapist and there are concerns about their constant accessibility leaving people at risk of becoming dependent on them – people aren't used to having a companion, even an AI one, constantly available to them, and always willing to offer friendly, positive and affirming comments. The draw can be too strong, and some experts are concerned that vulnerable people could end up communicating with them excessively in a bid to find comfort and reassurance.

Psychiatrists have also raised concerns that AI therapists lack emotional intelligence, and the cultural and social understanding human therapists have. This leaves them wanting as it means they can only rely on what you tell them whereas a psychiatrist or psychologist can pick up a lot of valuable information from observing things like your appearance, clothes and demeanour.[4] So, for example, you could tell your AI therapist that you're doing very well and there's no need for concern, whereas a human might spot that, despite your positive comments, you look exhausted, dishevelled and have lost a lot of weight. In this case, the human would adjust their treatment accordingly whereas the chatbot would be none the wiser and you could miss out on crucial interventions.

It seems some people are turning to AI chatbots for therapy while on waiting lists for real therapy and are finding them helpful – one 2025 study found that anxiety reduced by between thirty and thirty-five percent in people using AI therapy, compared with between forty-five and fifty percent in a group seeing human therapists[5] – but experts urge caution as there are few safeguards, and privacy can be an issue. These apps can collect large volumes of data and you may be unaware of exactly how it will be used.[6]

There is also a concern that these chatbots are programmed to be agreeable and so they can support bad ideas. For example, psychiatrists worry that were a person to tell a chatbot that they were thinking about ending their life, it might agree and tell them it was a good idea[7] because they are programmed to tell you what you want to hear and to take cues from what you say.

So, the long and the short of it is that AI therapists can provide some reassurance and immediately accessible guidance but it's not time to give up on the old-fashioned humans quite yet.

Having learned all of this, I decided to give AI therapy a go. I selected a professional therapy approach with a basis in CBT and asked the 'therapist' to speak to me in a friendly and empathic manner. So far so good. I then took a full therapy session with the chatbot, essentially an initial discussion in which it asked about my challenges and then suggested a treatment programme. At that point, it started asking for my credit card details, so I decided my jaunt into the world of AI therapy was over. Definitely a lot cheaper than private CBT with a human but, nonetheless, I didn't feel inclined to hand over my bank details.

But what was it like? Well, the first thing that struck me was it felt a bit laborious having to type all my answers out. I found myself answering more briefly than I might otherwise have done, essentially because I couldn't be bothered with any more typing. That limitation – laziness on my part – I think would have restricted the depth of the discussion had I taken the treatment programme further.

Some of the chatbot's answers and questions were also quite long and I started skim reading them. Again, laziness on my part. Basically, I prefer a proper chat with a human to endless reading and typing. Maybe, also, knowing I was communicating with a computer, not a person, made me less engaged in the conversation, or less respectful of the 'therapist's' insights – they held less value for me than had they come from a real therapist, so I was less inclined towards attending to them.

I suspect that on some apps you can probably get around the typing problem by using voice recognition and talking to the chatbot. I'm not sure this is particularly practical, though, because it would restrict use of the service to times when you're somewhere private – and this kind of defeats the object of a therapist that is constantly available. Unless, that is, you feel comfortable chatting about the ins and outs of your mental health to your phone on trains and the like...

So, putting aside my indolence, was the therapy any good? I will admit that the chatbot's questions and answers were sensible and well informed. It did mirror back to me what I'd said, and I might have wanted to kick its bank of stock responses after a while (think 'that's really understandable', 'that sounds really tough' and 'thank you for sharing that') but it also added respectable insights and asked appropriate questions.

The chatbot did, also, seem to know the fundamentals of emetophobia treatment – I couldn't fault anything it said for factual accuracy. For example, it advised me to try challenging my anxieties around food, telling me that going outside my comfort zone could help break the cycle of anxious thoughts. It told me that setting myself small challenges is key to overcoming my emetophobia and that doing so can help build confidence. It even explained that this approach is known as exposure.[8]

I think what it boiled down to for me was that I just don't

really want to spend my time chatting to a computer. To me, that is utterly depressing. To be engaged in a conversation, I need to be conversing with a person. Call me old fashioned but...

This tool was more like an extra-accessible Google – it could summarise in a simple and easily digestible form everything I could learn by googling 'emetophobia treatment', but it wasn't a therapist because therapy requires a human connection.

My top tips for protecting yourself in the digital world

And so, to my tips for protecting yourself online:

- Get your information from reliable online sources – a well-known mental health charity, such as Mind in the UK or the Anxiety and Depression Association of America, will offer accurate content which you can trust. This isn't necessarily true of posts by Joe Bloggs on TikTok...

- Avoid reading or watching content that triggers emetophobic thoughts – you know, don't read the articles about food recalls, salmonella outbreaks, and norovirus taking out hospitals. It isn't helpful to you when you read them. It's also ongoingly unhelpful as it teaches algorithms that you are interested in these stories and so you see more of them.

- Keep off forums and emetophobia groups. While they

can offer some understanding and support, they are awash with panic, anxiety and negativity that isn't what you need in your life.

- Where possible, interact with people in person, not online.
- Don't fall for people selling miracle cures online – sadly, there's no such thing.
- Be mindful of your use of social media – at least give some thought to whether it's serving you...or whether it is, in fact, toxic.
- While AI therapy is cheap, available 24/7 and has some value, don't rely on it as an alternative to a human therapist, especially if you are in a crisis.

Chapter 7

HOW ON EARTH IS THIS THING TREATED?

Right. Crunch time. We've looked at what emetophobia is, who has it, what causes it, and how it impacts people's lives. But, and it's a big but, so far, we've only looked at how to live with emetophobia. So, now for the crucial question: how do we get to the point of living without it? In other words, how on earth is this thing treated?

Diagnosis...or misdiagnosis

Before your emetophobia can be successfully treated, you need to know what it is you're living with. Now, I'm going to assume your emetophobia has been diagnosed, or at least that you have self-diagnosed. If you didn't know what the problem was, you wouldn't be reading this book, would you? However, we should cover this briefly just in case...

Few people, including medical professionals, have heard of emetophobia or know its symptoms. This means it can be hard to get a diagnosis. It's frequently misdiagnosed as generalised anxiety disorder, OCD or an eating disorder. However, the treatment is very different, especially for eating disorders, so it's crucial to get an accurate diagnosis before you go any further. Misdiagnosis can end in receiving unsuccessful treatment and so losing faith in therapists.[1] This is disastrous if it stops you getting the treatment you need for your emetophobia. So, if you don't agree with the diagnosis you're given initially, don't be afraid to challenge it or to look for a second opinion – you will know if the diagnosis feels right and fits your symptoms.

Let's be honest, most people with emetophobia can self-diagnose – it doesn't take much more than glancing down a list of typical emetophobia symptoms. I remember clearly the first time I saw the symptoms of the phobia – I couldn't believe how closely they fitted my experience.

However, to be formally diagnosed, you must see a professional. To help them make a diagnosis they will probably ask you to explain the history of your anxiety and ask a series of questions. These might include questions about whether you avoid situations that could result in vomiting and whether your fear impacts your quality of life.[2]

I hope that you'll have an enlightened therapist who is aware of emetophobia and how severe it is. If so, it will be immediately obvious to them that you have the condition and require treatment. Once you've got a diagnosis, it's time to crack on with beating this thing.

If, however, you seek a diagnosis but don't get one, or you get one but don't think it's accurate, don't give up. Look for a second opinion. Fight your corner. It's crucial to have an accurate diagnosis so if that means seeing three different doctors, do it!

Ellie was lucky. As soon as she developed symptoms of emetophobia, her parents started researching them and worked out what was wrong with her and what treatment she needed.

Ellie explained, 'Initially my family and I were confused – we didn't know what it was – but my mum did loads of research and got me started on treatment very fast. I was so scared of eating anything. I had this obsession that I wouldn't eat anything at all. That was where I realised I had a big problem and needed treatment.'

Treatment

Okay, so you've got a diagnosis. An accurate one, that is. What now?

Therapists Dr David Russ and Anna Christie say, 'Even though emetophobia is a terribly debilitating condition, it is highly treatable. Thousands of clinicians are now treating emetophobia very successfully and tens of thousands of people with emetophobia are finding healing and a new lease of life.'[3]

You see, it requires dedication and hard work, but it is doable.

There are really two options – either you buy a CBT workbook (see Further Reading) and work through it yourself, or you find a therapist who will help you. In all honesty, it's better if you can find a good therapist, as you will benefit from another person's support, guidance, encouragement and expertise. However, if you don't have access to therapy – it can be very expensive and there are often long waiting lists – and you are sufficiently determined, you can achieve the same recovery on your own.

How do I find a therapist?

So, I've said that in an ideal world you would work through your emetophobia treatment with the help of a therapist. But where do you find one? Especially a good one who is familiar with treating this condition?

The answer is that it varies from one country to another. In the UK, your GP is usually a good place to start. They will be aware of what mental health services are available in your area and can refer you. This strategy has the distinct advantage that it's free on the NHS. The downside is that there's often a very long waiting list for treatment; indeed, if you aren't deemed seriously unwell, you may find you never get to the top of the list.

If you don't want to see your GP in person, you may be eligible to self-refer to the NHS's Child and Adolescent Mental Health Services (CAMHS). This is a free service aimed at helping young people access mental health support from counsellors, psychiatrists, mental health nurses and psychologists. Some patients require a referral from their GP; others can self-refer. Check out the website of your local CAMHS for details.

The alternative is to look for a private therapist. This way you usually don't have to wait for treatment to begin and can choose which therapist you want to see. The downsides of this strategy are that they can be very expensive and aren't always as well regulated as NHS therapists. To get round this, try looking for a therapist on the website of the British Association for Behavioural and Cognitive Psychotherapies.[4] Any therapist you find on that site is accredited and, therefore, more reliable. You would still need to check, though, what experience they have with treating emetophobia specifically. Another option is the British Association for Counselling and Psychotherapy (BACP)[5] which keeps a register of counsellors who meet a recommended set of quality standards, or the United Kingdom Council for Psychotherapy's (UKCP) 'Find a therapist' tool which can help you search therapists who are fully qualified.[6]

Things are a bit different in the US and Canada. Emetophobia expert Anna Christie's website, Emetophobia Help,[7] has a list of therapists in the USA and Canada who treat emetophobia – you could try checking out this list to see if she recommends a therapist near you. If not, Anna recommends visiting the Psychology Today website[8] and using the 'Find a Therapist' tool to locate someone local to you who treats emetophobia. You would either have to self-fund your treatment or go through your insurance provider.

Therapy – CBT

Going to see a therapist for the first time is a huge step – it can feel terrifying. Don't worry – the therapists know this too. Dr Russ and Anna Christie have written a book for therapists on how to treat emetophobia. It's called *Emetophobia: Understanding and Treating Fear of Vomiting in Children and Adults*. They tell therapists that their patients are likely to be 'desperate, courageous and terrified'. They explain they'll be, 'Desperate because this fear is so debilitating. Courageous because the very act of coming for help is threatening. Terrified because they know they will need to talk about and potentially face the very thing that is so horrifying they will do nearly anything to escape it.'[9]

So, hopefully the therapist will be empathetic but what will you have to do in therapy? Well, the generally recognised treatment for emetophobia is CBT with exposure therapy. The CBT is essentially a way of teaching you how to help yourself and is effective regardless of what triggered the emetophobia – it focuses on what is happening now, rather than on past trauma.[10] So, no lying on a sofa delving into childhood traumas or your relationship with your mother. It involves working with how you think (that's the cognitive bit) and how you behave (that's the behavioural bit) and learning to question and shift them gently in a healthier direction.

People with emetophobia tend to believe vomiting is the worst thing that can possibly happen, and that if they're sick, they will be completely unable to cope with it. CBT for emetophobia involves working on shifting that belief to an understanding that, while it isn't pleasant, vomiting is not the worst thing imaginable and is something you could cope with.[11] Once that shift in understanding has been achieved, shaking off safety-seeking behaviours and avoidance tactics is much easier – they're no longer needed.

Having CBT for emetophobia generally also involves setting goals of things you would like to achieve that you aren't currently able to because of your emetophobia.[12] These could include going out to eat at your local restaurant, going on holiday, or going to stay overnight at a friend's house – whatever is important to you. These goals give you something positive to work towards and act as motivation to stay focused on your treatment.

Another common exercise in CBT involves considering the pros and cons of recovery. You might be asked to write a list of the pros of recovering from your emetophobia, such as being able to visit relatives in hospital, being able to go out for lunch with your friends or being able to give a presentation. You may then be asked to write a list of the cons, such as feeling increased anxiety and having to give up behaviours that have made you feel safer.[13] You can then work through your lists with your therapist. You might discuss whether the exercise has made you think it's worth tackling your emetophobia despite the possible challenges involved. After all, you're much more likely to stick with the treatment plan if you know exactly why you're doing it.

Ellie said, 'Emetophobia had taken over my life, so treatment was hard at first, but it got easier as I went through the process. I had CBT and exposure therapy. The CBT really helped a lot. I deal with situations a lot better now. I've learned how to calm myself down. I'm so much better now – I handle things completely differently.'

Therapy – exposure

Before we go into this, let me be very clear about one thing: exposure therapy for emetophobia never requires the person to be sick. That would be unethical and isn't necessary for successful treatment. It isn't relevant anyway because in people with emetophobia the problem isn't the vomiting, it's the anxiety.[14]

Once you've used CBT to think through why you're doing it and to start retraining your brain, your therapist is likely to introduce exposure therapy. There are two strands to it – exposure to increasingly graphic images and videos of people being sick, and exposure to foods, activities and situations that make you anxious. It also requires you to take on these challenges without relying on any of your safety-seeking behaviours. So, for example, you may be required to go to a restaurant and eat a full meal without first checking the establishment's food hygiene rating or taking any anti-nausea medication.

Unfortunately, the reality of emetophobia treatment is that if you want to beat your anxiety, you have to experience it – you must challenge yourself to do things that make you anxious and nauseous, so you learn they are, in fact, safe.[15] So, for therapy to be successful you really have to work hard on the homework assignments and be dedicated to doing them week after week.

Since I've been well enough to engage with it, I've twice had brief spells of CBT for my emetophobia and, I'll be honest, I didn't make any real effort with the homework challenges so, surprise, surprise, I didn't get better. If I'm looking to make excuses, I'd say my therapist was too nice – I knew it wouldn't be picked up on if I hadn't done them, so I didn't try. But, if I now put on my adult hat, I should have done them anyway for my own benefit. I was just cheating myself. I guess I just wasn't sufficiently motivated to do them. That and not committed enough, or brave enough. And that's why I still have emetophobia symptoms and avoidance behaviours. Maybe it was also partly arrogance on my part – I didn't believe it would help me. More fool me, is all I can say. Ellie is proof of how effective the treatment is if engaged with properly.

Zoe has tried lots of different treatments, including CBT and hypnotherapy. She said, 'I realised I had a problem when I thought about how much time I spent thinking about vomiting. It makes me sad. I mean, every night I go to bed hoping nothing will happen in the night.'

She continued, 'The emetophobia is a feeling of lack of control and it makes me feel like I'm going to crumble and that it'd be a catastrophe. The treatment helped me to build my confidence and self-esteem, and it helped me accept that I can't control everything. It aimed to help me better control my thoughts and feelings because you can't control anything else.'

Ellie also had exposure therapy. She said, 'I went to exposure and that helped a lot. It was probably one of the hardest things I've ever done, but it was definitely the best thing I've ever done. I had a year of treatment and emetophobia just isn't a major problem that I have any more.'

Ellie explained that as part of the exposure therapy she had to gradually start trying different foods and, also, gradually start building back up to going to school. For example, she was anxious about getting the school bus, so she started by being dropped off by her parents and progressed to getting the bus when she was feeling more confident.

Throughout exposure therapy you should always be in control – it should go at a pace you're comfortable with, there shouldn't be any surprises, and you should be able to stick with each level of exposure for as long as you need before moving on to the next.[16] If you feel that your therapist is putting too much pressure on you, or going too fast, you're well within your rights to ask them to slow down. In fact, you should do that because the treatment is more likely to be successful if you fully master each stage before moving on to the next.

Right, so let's look at exposure in more detail. First, treatment involves eventually learning to cope with seeing people being sick. So, in therapy, a person with emetophobia will be required initially to look at, say, the word vomit, then cartoon images of someone looking a bit nauseous. Once they can do that comfortably, it will build up to cartoons of someone being sick, then photos of real people feeling unwell, being sick and so on. Eventually, they will be asked to watch videos of people being sick, maybe first with the sound off and then, eventually, with it on.

I should explain, also, it isn't a case of just glancing at each of these pictures or clips once – it requires daily exposure to them for, maybe, twenty minutes at a time, until you can watch them over and over without any anxiety or repulsion.

I can see why this works. When I was a teenager, if the dog was sick I got extremely anxious and ran a mile, but after years of living with dogs and their sometimes-unsavoury habits, I'm now pretty relaxed about my dogs throwing up. Exposure therapy, isn't it? Normalisation.

Alongside exposure to people being sick, a person in treatment for emetophobia is also required to challenge their anxious and avoidant behaviours and to gradually start doing all the things their emetophobic voice tells them not to. Examples could include travelling on public transport, eating chicken, going on a boat, drinking alcohol or spending time around drunk people in a pub.

The purpose of this is to teach your brain that these activities are, in fact, perfectly safe and that you will come to no harm from doing them. The more times you do something and aren't sick, the more you prove to yourself that you can do it. Just doing it once isn't enough, I'm afraid, because that can leave you feeling you just got lucky and got away with it that once. It must be done repeatedly until it becomes normal and anxiety-free for you.[17]

On the off chance that you actually are sick, well, part of the purpose of CBT for emetophobia is learning to accept that occasionally people do vomit but that it doesn't matter any more than getting the occasional cold matters. If you were sick, the chances are you would just see for yourself that it's a perfectly manageable experience and that the people around you would likely be nothing but kind and caring.

I'm going to use an analogy – I love them, after all, so humour me here. If a child is afraid of jumping into a pool and they keep avoiding it, they will never learn that it's fun, and safe. If they bravely give it a go just once, while screaming and clinging onto a parent's hand, they have tried it, which is great, but they still haven't got over their fear. Have you ever watched a child try something like this? Well, what happens next? They try it a few more times, right? Maybe while holding a float initially. And then within a few minutes they are jumping in again and again, squealing with delight and wondering why they were ever so scared because it's great fun. Emetophobia exposure challenges are essentially the same. Practise enough and you'll be skipping into that fried chicken shop declaring that it's your new favourite dinner spot!

Importantly, while undertaking exposure challenges for emetophobia, no safety-seeking behaviours are permitted as they undermine the legitimacy of the challenge. So, no asking for reassurance that food is fully cooked, no overcooking food, asking other people how they're feeling, checking expiration dates, scanning rooms for the nearest bathroom or excessive handwashing.[18] To extend the swimming pool analogy, if the child will only jump in with a float to hand, they haven't escaped their fear. Assuming they can swim competently, they're only free of the fear once they're jumping in happily without a float anywhere in sight.

This is a bit grim, I must say, but some therapists also require patients to make some fake vomit – I don't know, parmesan soup or something – and to look at it poured in a loo, or to tip it all over the floor and then practise clearing it up. The reason for this is that many people with emetophobia feel they wouldn't be able to cope with tidying up after someone had been sick. This exercise involves normalising this process.

The research shows that the more a patient challenges themselves, exposes themselves to things that make them anxious, and the more difficult the challenges they set themselves, the greater and quicker their recovery will be. However, it is also understood that most people with emetophobia, me included, are very reluctant to engage in CBT with exposure. Catch 22.

This is the crux of the problem: the treatment requires complete buy-in from the patient – you need to be up for challenging yourself every single day – however, most people with the phobia aren't willing to do so because they aren't willing to take what they perceive to be a huge risk. This applies even for adults who are actively seeking treatment for themselves. It's even worse if teenagers or young people are forced to attend therapy by well-meaning parents – if you don't want to be there, what are your chances of throwing yourself into the challenges? Extremely low, I would say. Certainly, dragging me to therapy when I was a teenager would have achieved nothing. It's the jumping out of a plane without a parachute thing again. If you view your emetophobia as your parachute, you aren't going to want to lose it, however much suffering it is causing you.

However, if you can, it is so worth working through a structured and manageable programme of exposures because they are the key to recovery. To get your life back, you need to commit to them. The more you do, the better you will get and the less you will feel a need for the metaphorical parachute – you will learn that you aren't actually jumping out of a plane at all. And it needn't be too scary – you can, and should, go at a speed you are comfortable with, doing exposures that challenge you but don't terrify or upset you. Be brave – you will reap the rewards.

Another treatment option that some people find helpful is known as imagery re-scripting.[19] This is particularly relevant if your emetophobia was triggered by an upsetting experience. It involves talking through the experience in detail to relive it. It then requires you to identify what would have made the situation less traumatic and to re-imagine it with that change made in your mind. For example, if you were abandoned when you were ill, you could re-imagine the experience with your adult self there to look after and support your younger self.

Overall, it's thought that, on average, it takes about two to three years to rewire an emetophobic brain to more healthy thinking, but this requires consistency, sticking with therapy until the end of the course, and completing homework assignments.[20] As with so many things in life, the more you put in, the more you get out – the harder you work on your homework challenges, the more successful you will be in overcoming your emetophobia. The eventual aim is to rewire your brain, so your thoughts naturally head down healthy pathways, not emetophobic ones.

Ellie said, 'I can't remember the last time I was worried about being sick. I wouldn't panic about it any more and I don't think about it all the time any more. That fear no longer impacts my life.

'I would recommend exposure therapy one hundred percent to anyone with emetophobia. It sorted it out for me and I got so much better.'

Here I need to add a word of caution, or of realism. It isn't always possible to completely cure people with emetophobia. Many, me included, will retain some of the habits, worries and behaviours associated with the phobia. Don't be downhearted by this, though, because almost everyone with the condition can improve significantly. They can improve enough that their quality of life is transformed. They can get to a place where their emetophobia no longer controls them and causes them daily distress.

It's about momentum not perfection. Part of the underlying issue with emetophobia can be a desire to obsessively control everything. Part of successful treatment is accepting that there are elements of ourselves and the world around us that we cannot fully control and which won't be 'perfect' – that is not to say that you can't have a rich fulfilling life that is no longer dominated by the condition.

Dr Keyes and Professor Veale treat people with emetophobia day in, day out. They say, 'Not everyone can be "cured" of emetophobia, but they are able to recover the parts of their lives that they feel they have missed out on. They may still have some fears of vomiting but no longer feel restricted.'[21]

How can my friends and family help me overcome my emetophobia?

Chances are that your closest friends and family, particularly your parents if you live with them, will want to understand your emetophobia and to help you if they can. But how do you help them to help you?

First, they can't help if they don't know what's happening, so you need to educate them. I know it can be hard to be open about your emetophobia, and that you may feel ashamed, or fear being misunderstood or judged, but the potential benefits are huge. So, if you can, start by explaining what's going on in your head and give them some emetophobia intel. You could consider giving them a copy of this book or could direct them to other reputable sources of information. The more they understand, the better placed they will be to support you.

You could also explain that what you need is for them to provide patient emotional support as well as encouragement and motivation to keep going with treatment.[22] They will probably find it empowering to be given a helpful role like this – caring for someone with emetophobia can make people feel helpless so having a clear brief of how to help can make them feel better too.

The major challenge to be aware of is that you don't allow those around you to help perpetuate your fear – seeking reassurance from them is a form of safety-seeking behaviour and, while those make you feel better in the short term, they keep the fear going in the long run. So, the ideal supportive person, whoever they may be, will offer emotional support in the form of a hug or a listening ear, but they won't offer reassurance.[23]

For example, if you're worried your supper is undercooked, they won't tell you that it's very well cooked and safe to eat, but might instead make you a cup of tea and encourage you, kindly, to challenge yourself and just eat it. Explain that for your recovery, this is the role you need them to play. It may also be worth being clear that they mustn't push you to go too fast, or too far, out of your comfort zone. It must be done at your pace. Over-enthusiastic attempts to plough through and get you 'cured' as fast as possible won't help anyone.

While it's undoubtedly helpful to explain all of this to your nearest and dearest, it's best to do it when you are calm and balanced. In that frame of mind, you can lay all this out clearly and rationally. Let's be honest, if you raise it when you're already feeling anxious, you'll find it much more difficult to insist that they don't reassure you!

It might also help to explain that if your behaviour is sometimes challenging, or extreme – you know, if you throw tantrums, basically – the reason is that you are being forced to do something that makes you very anxious. When adults have emetophobia, they generally just avoid things that make them anxious. This can be harder for children and teens because parents and teachers may force them to do things. This can make them feel trapped and panicked and out of control, resulting in 'bad' behaviour.[24] If you explain the reason why you are behaving in a certain way, you can much better work through it together with compassion rather than with a caregiver who just thinks discipline is required.

You could ask a parent or guardian to attend therapy with you. Depending on your age, the therapist might ask that you do this. This adult can then be educated as to how best to help you and can act as an unofficial therapist outside the sessions.

Medication

Almost everyone with emetophobia requires CBT and exposure therapy to overcome the condition – there's no quick fix, sadly, and you can't dodge the hard work. However, there's another treatment tool for emetophobia which can help and which, in fact, was the key to my own recovery. Medication.

Many people with emetophobia are wary of taking medication, you guessed it, for fear it makes them sick. Also, because they have concerns about side effects, withdrawal symptoms, dependency and having their 'mind altered'. However, medication can be life-changing, even lifesaving. So read on...

Technically there are no medications licensed for the treatment of emetophobia;[25] however, antidepressants and anti-anxiety medications are often recommended to people with emetophobia with particularly severe symptoms, or those who are so anxious they're unable to take part in the exposure therapy.[26] In these cases, medication can help them take part actively in therapy. Medication can be particularly helpful for people with strong OCD tendencies as part of their emetophobia.[27]

In my case, I'm sure being prescribed a selective serotonin reuptake inhibitor (SSRI) for my acute anxiety while I was on my gap year was the turning point in my experience of emetophobia. I'm quite sure that without it I wouldn't have been able to go to university or to lead a 'normal' student life. In fact, I don't think I could have started making any progress with treating my emetophobia because, until I was on the SSRI, I didn't want to get better.

These medications can be prescribed by your doctor, or by a psychiatrist, but not by a counsellor or psychologist. You should be aware that they require patience because it can take up to four weeks to see any improvement, and as long as sixteen weeks to get the full benefits[28] – as with all emetophobia treatments, they're not a quick fix.

If you and your doctor decide to go down this route, there are a few different SSRIs that can be tried. These include citalopram, escitalopram, sertraline and fluoxetine and several others.[29] Which one you're prescribed initially will depend on various factors, including your specific symptoms and your age. In some cases, people find they don't get on with the first one they try and so need to try a few to find the one that works best for them.

The main downside of taking these meds is that they can come with a range of side effects. No one gets all of them. Some people get none. Which you get, if any, may depend on which drug you are taking and on the dose. Most of the possible side effects, such as nausea, fatigue, headaches, a dry mouth and excessive sweating, wear off after a couple of weeks.[30] What it boils down to is do the side effects of the medications outweigh the benefits of taking them? That's something you can only find out by trying.

For me, the SSRI did cause side effects for the first week or two, as I will explain in a minute, but those rapidly wore off. The only lasting side effects I had from it were occasional night sweats and sleepiness but those were only a problem when I was taking very high doses. On lower doses, the benefits absolutely outweighed the downsides, no doubt about it.

It is generally accepted that SSRIs are just as effective as CBT for the treatment of OCD, so the evidence is in their favour for emetophobia treatment as almost everyone with emetophobia experiences symptoms of OCD.

The amount of information available and the range of different perspectives among experts makes it a tricky and controversial subject. All I can suggest is that you talk to your doctor or psychiatrist. Then you can make an informed decision about what is best for you.

So, if you decide to take the plunge and try the meds, the first question many people ask is, how long would you need to be on them? Well, that varies hugely from one person to another, on the rate of your recovery, and on your general mental wellbeing, but it's generally thought that you should stay on them until you've been fully recovered for a couple of years, and for at least six months after finishing CBT. This is to give you a chance to really solidify your recovery before losing that support.[31]

If you decide to come off them, especially if you've been taking them for a while, it's advisable to do it very gradually and in discussion with your doctor. This is to reduce the likelihood of withdrawal symptoms and relapse. So, for example, if you're on 20mg you might reduce it to 10mg for a few months and see how you get on before cutting it completely.

Even with these precautions, you may experience short-lived withdrawal symptoms. Again, there are various possible symptoms, and they vary from person to person, but they can include dizziness, agitation and insomnia.[32] Some people also describe an electric-shock-type sensation as the nerve synapses react to losing the SSRI. I felt this in my chest and a friend in her head. Again, it generally disappears after a week or two and it's not dangerous – it just feels a bit odd.

I can reassure you that, while withdrawal symptoms can make coming off SSRIs tricky, these medications are not addictive. Many people are reluctant to take them for fear of becoming dependent on them, but this shouldn't be too much of a concern.

It's usually straightforward getting a prescription for SSRIs if you want to try them and your doctor agrees you need them, and they might help you.

* * *

So that's SSRIs. The other type of medication most commonly discussed in emetophobia literature is antiemetics – anti-sickness drugs. These are a completely different ball game because they're sometimes used by people with emetophobia as a means of controlling their nausea or trying to reduce the chance of vomiting. Basically, they're taken as a safety-seeking behaviour. As a result, people with emetophobia often request these medications. However, while they may have a placebo effect, they don't technically work on anxiety-induced nausea so are of no benefit in the treatment of emetophobia.[33] Indeed, they may be counterproductive because, as we've learned, for recovery it's crucial people with emetophobia give up their safety-seeking behaviours. So, for example, if someone takes on the exposure challenges but then downs a load of antiemetics afterwards, they've cheated, and the exposure therapy won't be successful.

Far from being used as an emetophobia treatment, antiemetics should, in fact, be gradually stopped as part of treatment if someone is taking them regularly.[34] Sorry!

* * *

Some people with emetophobia are prescribed anxiolytics – anti-anxiety drugs – to be used in particularly difficult moments, such as if they are having a panic attack. These can sometimes be helpful if only taken very occasionally and in extreme circumstances. For example, if you had to get on a boat and the idea was making you extremely panicked. Generally, therapists treating people with emetophobia are not keen on them having anxiolytics because they are also often used as a safety-seeking behaviour and we know how much therapists like those![35]

My experience

The big turning point in my experience of emetophobia came in February of my gap year, when I turned nineteen. This birthday was significant for one reason: for years the doctor had refused to give me antidepressants on the grounds I was too young. After my birthday, medication became an option.

I was torn about whether I wanted to take it. I was afraid of how it would make me feel, whether I would become dependent on it and, of course, of the possible side effects. I was also aware I'd been suffering for years and that it was only a matter of months until I was due to start at university and I wasn't well enough. I didn't really have a choice. These meds were my best chance of making it to university. So, I accepted the prescription, forced myself not to look at the list of side effects, and downed the first dose before I could change my mind.

The doctor had been very clear that, especially as I was still a teenager, I would have to go and see him once a week initially, and that I was to ring him immediately if I had any problems with the meds.

So, what happened when I went on them? Well, the morning after I started taking the antidepressants, I started to notice the early side effects. It was extremely difficult to wake up. Though, to be fair, getting up in the morning has never been a strong point of mine. My body felt like it was made of lead. It had no interest in moving an inch. I just wanted to lie motionless and sleep.

Something else also felt different. I was lying sprawled out on my back in bed, like a starfish. Usually, I woke curled up in a tight ball, tense and trying to shield myself from the world. On this occasion, I felt relaxed in my spreadeagled pose and had none of my normal manic energy. I lay staring at the ceiling and enjoying the stillness and heaviness of my unusually calm body.

My mind, also, was empty. No anxious thoughts. Sort of a void. Maybe one that was filled with cottonwool. Nothing going on in there. That was easy enough to handle. Good.

Thirty mindless, inactive minutes later, I employed all the willpower I could muster and dragged myself out of bed. In the kitchen I noticed Mum was about to start unloading the dishwasher. I was a teenager, right? Usually, if I'm honest, I'd have left her to empty it while I made my own breakfast, lost in my thoughts. But on this day, something was different. I felt a sort of gentle compulsion to help her. I wandered over and started unloading the dishwasher. Turned out, doing the dishwasher is quick and easy and that Mum appreciated the help.

How could a little white pill suddenly make me feel inclined towards helping Mum in the kitchen? Maybe it would be helpful to me? I certainly felt calm. Not anxious. And my body felt at peace, if somewhat leaden. It was only as I went to walk the dog that I noticed I was starting to feel a bit nauseous. Different nauseous, that is. Not the anxious queasiness I was used to. Maybe this was another side effect?

I reassured myself that these side effects wouldn't last long and continued to look out for positive signs in myself. Once some of the initial terror of taking the medication had faded, I started to enjoy spotting tiny shifts in myself. It was like a game of Spot the Difference but with my own inner self.

For a few days I existed in a twilight world. My brain felt like mush, my body like a block of lead. Waves of gentle nausea washed over me. I had no appetite and all I wanted to do was lie around in my pyjamas.

This state wasn't unpleasant, really. At least, not compared to what I was used to. It was calm and restful and undemanding. A welcome break from anxiety and highly strung energy. From an adrenaline-fuelled existence. I was grateful not to have the energy to worry. The funny thing is that I felt a bit sick, but I wasn't worried about it. The citalopram had kind of turned the dial down on the anxiety.

This state wasn't unpleasant because I wasn't being required to do anything. I was free to indulge it. It would've been a completely different matter if I'd had to go to school or work. In fact, I don't think I could have. I didn't feel well enough. Not enough mental or physical 'umph'.

However, as the days went by, I gradually started to feel better. The nausea started to subside, I felt up for being out and about again and my brain slowly regained its functionality.

As my brain reawakened, I noticed it felt a little different. I felt lighter, more upbeat and positive. I suddenly felt an interest in looking after myself, in nurturing myself and in trying to improve my health and wellbeing. I felt motivated to make positive changes. The apathy and self-destructiveness had gone. It suddenly felt important to heal myself, and as though that might be possible. How could one tiny pill achieve all this? How could it change my thoughts so profoundly? Regardless, this was crucial because it meant I was finally able to engage with the other elements of emetophobia treatment.

It shocks me now that I ever lost interest in looking after myself. That I had reached a point where I no longer cared at all about my own wellbeing or felt any interest in attempting to improve it. I'm so grateful for the SSRIs because they opened this door and gave me the motivation and inclination to work on my recovery. Without the hope they allowed me to feel, I can't see how I could ever have started to get better.

Not only did the medication put an end to the self-destructiveness, but it also helped me to relax slightly around food. Suddenly, foods that had previously been off the menu seemed more manageable and my anxiety around throwing up became slightly less intense. It certainly didn't cure my emetophobia, but it made it easier to live with. To live 'normally' with. It took the edge off it and meant I could start to nourish my body properly with a reasonably healthy and balanced, if restricted, diet.

It also reduced my anxiety sufficiently that I could once again do simple things like going to the pub with friends in the evening or sitting in a cinema. And all these little changes created something of a positive upwards cycle – having a healthier diet and being able to have fun with my friends were, in themselves, medicines. They were good for my health, both physical and mental, and helped with the slow but steady improvement in my wellbeing. I still credit the SSRIs with that.

That was my experience. Everyone is different but I hope this shows that, while going on medication can be frightening initially, it can also be well worth taking the plunge. I should add that I know people who have gone on it and not experienced any side effects at all. I took it throughout my time at university and for a year or so after I left but then I gradually came off it and was okay without it. So, don't worry, if you go on it, you won't be stuck on it for life. And remember, it really isn't addictive.

Zoe is also on an SSRI. She said, 'I find it incredibly helpful. I can't know for sure if it's the medication or just me, but I feel like I'm a bit better and more positive. I feel more centred on it. It's miserable going on and off it but I think it takes the edge off the emetophobia – it gives me a little foot up. It definitely does its job.'

My top tips for overcoming emetophobia

Now, what are my top tips for treating and overcoming your emetophobia?

- Be realistic but optimistic. You aren't going to be cured overnight, but recovery is possible.

- Celebrate small wins but don't beat yourself up when it goes wrong. No one manages all the exposure challenges first time – just do your best. If you don't manage one of them, try something slightly easier and come back to the tricky one later – don't lose hope or get angry with yourself. Beating emetophobia is hard but you'll get there.

- Accept that some days exposures feel easier than others. Sometimes you'll feel robust and brave and up for the challenges, other times you'll be feeling fragile and vulnerable and taking on an exposure challenge will feel overwhelming. That's okay. Trust that if one day it's too difficult, it might be easier the next. I still occasionally have days when I'm feeling overwhelmed and I know it won't go well if I try to cook something I find more challenging. Usually, things have shifted by the next day.

- Be open minded about medication – it isn't for everyone, and not everyone needs it, but it can be life-changing.

- If you see a therapist that you don't like, or don't find helpful, don't give up – switch to a different one. The same applies to doctors and psychiatrists.

- Don't give up on therapy too soon and do your best with the homework assignments – if you don't do them, you won't improve.[36]

- Explain to friends and family how they can support you in your recovery. For example, your therapist may suggest that you ask them not to shield you from things that might make you anxious.

- Ditch the perfectionism – even if you don't achieve a full 'cure' for your emetophobia, every step forward, and every bit of progress, will improve your quality of life.

Chapter 8

THE CRUCIAL IMPORTANCE OF SELF-CARE

We've now looked at emetophobia treatment, but following a formal treatment programme isn't the only thing you can do to improve your wellbeing. Making minor changes to your lifestyle can also have a huge impact on your overall health. That's what we're going to consider in this chapter.

Self-care

I loathe the term self-care. It makes me cringe. Nonetheless, call it what you will, it's crucial. Of course, it's important all the time but it's particularly important when you have, or are trying to recover from, emetophobia. This is because looking after yourself is beneficial for your mental health so a bit of effort in this department will make overcoming your emetophobia easier – we all know we feel more cheerful and proactive if we've had plenty of sleep, and that a bit of exercise gives us an energy boost and the so called 'runner's high'. You see?

Dr Rangan Chatterjee, author of *The 4 Pillar Plan: How to Relax, Eat, Move, Sleep Your Way to a Longer, Healthier Life*, says, 'The right lifestyle and nutrition can actually improve our wellbeing, reverse our health problems and can even make chronic diseases like type 2 diabetes, obesity and depression disappear.'[1]

He adds, 'Good health occurs outside the doctor's surgery – not inside. Our lifestyles themselves are often the best medicine.'[2]

Self-care is also important for people with emetophobia because the healthier and more robust you feel physically, the better able you will be to tackle your emetophobia. If you wake up feeling exhausted, stressed and bloated from a night of binge-watching Netflix, drinking fizzy drinks and eating pizza, are you going to feel like taking on some tricky exposure challenges? Honestly, no, I don't think so. You're going to want to roll over in bed and go straight back to sleep, or to have a duvet day. Restful as those may be, they aren't going to cure you of your emetophobia. So, apologies about the tough love, but as part of getting better you need to look after all aspects of your health. It'll create a sort of positive cycle of all-round improvement. Don't sabotage yourself for the sake of another hour of TikTok, or a third Mars bar.

I could probably write a whole book on the topic of wellbeing and self-care – plenty of people have done. But don't worry, we're just going to do a whistlestop tour of the fundamentals in this chapter.

To get on top of your overall health there are four main areas we need to look at – diet, exercise, sleep and rest. Nurturing good relationships with friends and family is also a crucial part of wellbeing but I won't subject you to any more on that topic. We covered it in Chapter 4. The key with all of this is to experiment and see what works best for you – what fits in with your life and what makes you feel good.

Diet

Emetophobia can, as we know, have a huge impact on your ability to eat, and to nourish your body. We looked at the challenges of eating with emetophobia in Chapter 3. This chapter is for exploring what we would ideally eat for optimal health. It's something to aim for, and you will hopefully be able to make the general principles work for you even with the limitations of emetophobia.

While you may feel eating better won't make any difference to your mental health, the experts would beg to differ. A study in 2017, rather charmingly known as the SMILES trial, looked at the impact of switching people with severe depression to a Mediterranean-style diet high in fish, fruit, veggies and wholegrains. Incredibly, after three months, about a third of the patients on the diet were in remission. This compared to only eight percent in the control group.[3] So, while the research on the impact of diet on mental health is still in its infancy, it might just be well worth the effort.

So, what are these principles you might want to try adopting? Let's pull out some bullet points:

- Avoid processed food as much as possible. If it's in a packet and has a billion ingredients then, chances are, it's not good for you. If nothing else, half of those ingredients are probably sugar and random chemicals with names no one can pronounce. Are those likely to be good for you? Doubtful. If it needs no label, and is more or less as nature made it, then it's a go-er. So, avocados, eggs, apples and steak are good. Chocolate bars, breakfast cereals, muffins and protein bars, not so much.

- Avoid sugar. That omnipresent white stuff causes a blood sugar rollercoaster which leads to mood swings, energy peaks and troughs, cravings and anxiety. Simply by avoiding processed food you will slash your sugar intake – most processed foods are laden with it, even ones you wouldn't expect, like pasta sauces and yoghurts. Watch out for sugar in drinks too – fruit juices, smoothies, sodas, cocktails and the like are all full of it.

- Eat plenty of fruit and vegetables. It doesn't matter if they're dried, frozen, fresh, whatever. Just eat as many as you can (within reason) and aim for as much variety as possible. In fact, let's say plant foods, not just fruits and veg, so throw in as many nuts, seeds and beans as possible too. They're all fab for your microbiome as well as being packed with essential vitamins, minerals and fibre, not to mention some protein. They'll keep those gut bugs healthy, and the gut bugs will, in turn, make you healthy. Everyone wins. So top avocado toast with mixed seeds, snack on nuts, and finish meals with a piece of fruit.

- Make sure every meal has a sensible balance of high-quality protein, healthy carbs, good fats and veggies. That'll keep you well-nourished and your energy stable. For example, you might have some chicken breast (remember, this chapter is about what we are aiming to be able to eat...), salmon, cheese, eggs or chickpeas for your protein; sourdough bread (better for you than normal bread), brown rice, sweet potato or quinoa as your carb; avocado, nuts, olive oil or oily fish to pack in some healthy fats; and plenty of greens. I'll give you an example. For my lunch I just had sourdough toast (carb) with avocado (healthy fat), tomatoes (veg...okay, okay, I know they're technically fruits), mozzarella (protein), a drizzle of olive oil (healthy fat) and a sprinkle of mixed seeds (healthy fat and protein). I then added a couple more plant foods and some extra vitamins by having raspberries, a couple of squares of very dark chocolate, and a handful of nuts for dessert. Took five minutes to make, was packed full of goodness and was delicious.

So, those are the basics. All these principles apply whatever your dietary preferences – whether you are vegan, vegetarian, on a carnivore diet, have food allergies or anything else. Regardless of your personal preferences, a balanced diet of minimally processed whole foods is your best bet.

Of course, much as this idea upsets the perfectionist in me, no one is perfect, it's impossible to be perfect and perfection is a ridiculous thing to aim for. I know that logically, but... So, no need to stick to these principles all the time – most of the time is good enough. Yesterday was my son's seventh birthday. Was his cake a processed, sugary, chemical-filled health monstrosity? Of course! But did I have a slice (or three)? You bet I did!

Exercise

Love it, or hate it, exercise is crucial for your mental and physical wellbeing. It improves your immune system, your gut microbiome (yes, those little bugs again), your hormone balance, your circulation, your brain health, your mental wellbeing, your sleep and your blood pressure, among many other things. It also reduces your risk of cancer, diabetes, anxiety, depression and even of Alzheimer's in old age.[4]

Exercise is also known to be good for reducing anxiety. This is because, among other clever things, exercising causes the body to release endorphins, which create a feeling of general wellbeing. It also impacts other neurotransmitters such as serotonin and dopamine, which help regulate mood.

You get the idea – exercise is good for you. In all honesty, it doesn't really matter what you do, just do something. Ideally, a form of exercise that builds cardio fitness, one that works on muscle strength, and one that improves flexibility. So, for example, you could go running a couple of times a week, do weights in the gym a couple of times, and do a yoga session or two. The possibilities are endless. Try to find what works for you and, crucially, what you enjoy. Let's be honest, if you don't like it, you aren't going to stick to it.

As with food, don't worry about trying to be perfect. Everyone has some weeks where everything goes wrong, they're under the weather, injured, or they simply can't be bothered, and you may be too busy to fit much exercise in anyway – anything you can do will be beneficial. A fifteen-minute walk at lunchtime every day is great, so is a weekly parkrun, as is a game of cricket with some mates, or an evening yoga class. I did our local parkrun this morning – my time was very slow because my children ran one of the laps with me (that's my excuse, anyway) but that doesn't matter. The point is I got my body moving, raised my heartrate and worked up a bit of a sweat.

If you're short of time (or motivation) be clever and get as much out of each exercise session as possible. For example, a dynamic yoga class can work your muscles, your cardiovascular system, your balance and your flexibility. Or an interval training workout which includes squats and lunges can build muscle as well as cardio fitness.

For me, I know my dogs need walking every day, so I like to kill two self-care birds with one stone (sorry about the slightly morbid cliché) by going for a walk each morning with a friend, or with my mum, straight after dropping my children at school. I get some time chatting with a friend, an hour's gentle exercise, and the dogs get walked. How's that for efficient?!

It's my experience that the different areas of self-care link together in that, say, you do a yoga class, you are then more likely to feel like eating something healthy. My body is a temple kind of vibes. Or if you've eaten a really good breakfast, you're more likely to then feel energetic and to fancy going for a run. If, like me right now, you've eaten too much chocolate (still blaming my son's birthday), and you feel bloated and slightly sick, you aren't going to want to go and take some exercise. It's another example of a positive... or negative...feedback loop.

Sleep

Potentially a more appealing option than exercise, let's talk about sleep. Good sleep can improve your energy levels, your concentration, your stress levels, your mental health and even your life expectancy. Not only that, but when you've slept well, you're in with a much better chance of eating and exercising well too.[5] Another positive feedback loop!

Professor Matthew Walker, a sleep scientist who wrote a book called *Why We Sleep*,[6] says insufficient sleep has a signature in the brain very similar to stress. He says that when people don't get enough good quality sleep their levels of adrenaline, noradrenaline and cortisol all go up, as do their inflammation markers. As we know, these hormones are associated with anxiety, so we certainly don't need any more of them!

So how do you give yourself the best chance of a good night's sleep?

- Get up and go to bed at roughly the same time every day – yes, even at the weekend. This will set your body clock, or circadian rhythm as the experts call it, giving you a much better chance of falling asleep quickly and waking up refreshed.

- Keep your bedroom cool and as dark and quiet as possible. Install blackout blinds if necessary and turn off TVs, clocks, computers and any other devices that emit light. Even those tiny red ones are enough to impact your sleep quality.[7] We just got back from holiday, and the holiday house had green emergency escape route lights – all they achieved was keeping me awake every night!

- Make sure your mattress, pillows and bedding are comfortable and neither too heavy nor too light, so you aren't being disturbed by overheating, freezing or a sore back.

- Make yourself a bedtime routine. If you follow much the same routine every evening to wind down before trying to sleep – maybe a hot bath and then reading in bed – your body learns the cues and you're likely to get into bed already quite sleepy. I've always read a book in bed before going to sleep and my brain is now so effectively trained that reading is a cue to sleep – the mere sight of a book in the day is enough to see me nodding off... Not ideal for a writer!

- Don't stare at screens in the hour before you go to bed. The blue light emitted by phone, computer and iPad screens mimics that of morning light, sending a message to your brain that it's time to wake up. You're more likely to fall asleep quickly and to sleep well if you stick to relaxing, low lighting in the evenings.

- Try to get as much bright natural light and exercise as

you can in the morning. This helps with setting your body clock, so you feel perky in the day and sleepy by bedtime.

- Avoid alcohol. Even if it helps you fall asleep in the first place, it's well recognised that alcohol dramatically reduces the quality of your sleep, potentially without you even realising. It's best to avoid it altogether but if you want a drink, and are old enough to have one, try to have it earlier in the evening so it's out of your system by the time you go to sleep.

- Don't do anything crazy stressful just before you go to bed, like doom scroll social media feeds or look at all the changes your teacher wants made to your course-work. It just increases the chance that you'll lie in bed tossing and turning and fretting rather than sleeping.

- Go easy on the caffeine, especially in the afternoon.[8]

Rest

Bizarrely, rest is the self-care fundamental I find hardest. One would think it would be the easiest. I'm just not very good at sitting still. Thing is, though, that after all that exercise we're now doing (not to mention the emetophobia recovery), rest and relaxation are vital. De-stressing comes with a whole host of benefits from better sleep to improved emotional resilience.[9] Being chronically stressed is fairly disastrous for health – it's linked to increased risk of obesity, diabetes, high blood pressure, strokes, anxiety, depression and burnout.[10]

Indeed, it's thought that eighty per cent of all doctors' visits are linked to stress[11] in one way or another.

So, what are your options for relaxing and de-stressing? The list of possibilities is endless. Anything that you find restful and calming probably counts. You might even be able to tie in exercise with relaxation – a yoga class or a gentle walk somewhere beautiful can be very relaxing.

Alternatively, reading, meditation, massage, a hot bath, chatting to a friend, painting, knitting, sunbathing or listening to music are all good options – it's up to you! Whatever you choose, just try to find time for it every day, even if only for half an hour. That's enough to help you unwind a bit and to move you out of a stressed state and into a relaxed one.

There are other options you could also try for more active relaxation. You could try the meditations available on apps like Calm and Headspace, or you could give breathing exercises a go. For example, as we explored in Chapter 5, you could try so-called 'box breathing' or 3-4-5 breathing.[12] If you breathe slowly, you're telling your brain that you're in a calm state, and you will immediately feel less stressed.[13] It's the opposite of how you might hyperventilate when having a panic attack. Just a few minutes of breathing like this can make a tangible difference.

While these are all means of relaxing, it might also be wise to consider ways to reduce the amount of stress in your life. Think through your average day, putting aside your emetophobia – where is stress regularly coming from? Is there anything you can do to change it? For example, I know I feel stressed and flustered in the morning trying to get out of the door on time. What I should therefore do is get up ten minutes earlier. My stress level at the start of the day would be much lower were I to do this. Admittedly, even though I know this, I don't do it – that snooze button is just too tempting... What little changes could you make to reduce your stress levels?

My experience

When I was a young adult and first trying to recover from my emetophobia, I didn't know a whole lot about self-care. I mean, not more than the basics that everyone learns at school, from parents, common sense and the like. I'm not sure I was hugely interested in the topic either. I've become much more engaged with it as I've got older and so have only learned the benefits more recently. Now I'm very into it, am very conscientious about it, and am always reading books and listening to podcasts about health and wellbeing.

I'm constantly adjusting my lifestyle and diet to fit what's going on in my life and to try to make steady progress, but this is what I do currently:

- Try to eat primarily unprocessed, homecooked, whole foods. I don't eat any fast food, takeaways or ready meals. If I can make it organic and local I do but that's very difficult. I eat mainly plant foods but a little bit of meat and fish and quite a lot of eggs. Mainly, I focus on having masses of fruit, veg, nuts and seeds. My family would also report that I'm hopelessly addicted to dark chocolate.

- Take fish oils, vitamin D, probiotics and a multivitamin every day. I wouldn't take the fish oils if I ate more fish, but I know the fish oils EPA and DHA are crucial for brain health and I don't manage much fish.

- Walk my dogs for at least an hour every day, usually more, do a 5k run twice a week including our local parkrun on a Saturday, do a weights class in the neighbour's garden once a week, and horse riding three or four times a week. In a perfect world I would like to do weights twice a week (in fact, I wouldn't like to... I feel I ought to) and to do some yoga or Pilates because I'm astonishingly inflexible, but there just isn't time.

- Go to bed at 9pm every night and read until 10 or 10.30pm before going to sleep. No hardship, this one – I love my sleep! Rather harder is my aim to get up at 7am every day. Kicking myself out of bed is something I find a struggle, so that one tends to slip rather if I don't have to be up early.

- Keep alcohol consumption to a minimum and I don't smoke or take drugs.

That's where I'm at currently with what I've found best supports my health and wellbeing but I'm always up for learning more and making further improvements. I know I need to work on my stress levels. I'm sure they're unnecessarily through the roof. That's my next challenge!

My self-care top tips

- Eat as well as you can, as much of the time as you can, focusing on unprocessed, whole foods.

- Don't give up, feel guilty or get angry with yourself when it all goes wrong, you've gone to bed too late, eaten nothing but Haribo, and haven't got up off your sofa all day. Just calmly, and kindly, get yourself back on track – make the next meal healthy, go for a walk and go to bed early.

- Every little act of self-care, however small, will help. You don't need to run ultra-marathons (those are probably bad for you anyway) or live off kale – just do what feels manageable for you.

- Make self-care as enjoyable as possible. If you hate it, are forcing yourself to do it, and it makes you miserable then it probably isn't good for you. So, find things that are both good for your wellbeing, and that you enjoy. You'll then get the double benefit of the health boost and the enjoyment. For example, if you know you need to take more exercise, but you hate running and the gym, try playing tennis or football with friends or a dance class – still exercise but more fun!

- Prioritise your sleep. When you're contemplating whether to watch another twenty YouTube videos, pause for a moment to think which would serve you better – the epic fail videos or an extra hour's sleep.

- However busy you are, make time for at least half an hour's chilling every day. A soak in a hot bubble bath or reading a few pages of a favourite book is enough to send a message to your brain that everything is okay, and it can relax. You will reap rewards in all aspects of your life.

- If it all feels overwhelming, just make one small change at a time. For example, for the next week could you try going to bed an hour earlier? Or could you try adding an extra helping of vegetables at each meal? You don't have to tackle everything at once.

Chapter 9

LIFE AFTER EMETOPHOBIA

My experience

While this chapter is called Life after Emetophobia, in my case, at least, I think it would be more accurate to call it Life with the Dregs of Emetophobia.

Emetophobia no longer impacts my quality of life significantly. Well, I don't think it does, but I suppose I don't really know because I don't know what life is like for someone who has never had this phobia. Maybe it does still impact my quality of life. And perhaps it still has an impact on those around me – Jamie sometimes finds the legacy of it, and my ongoing control behaviours, stressful and frustrating. So maybe it does a bit. However, I think I can say it no longer controls my life, it no longer impacts my physical health, and it no longer causes me any notable suffering.

That's huge.

And, for me, I think it's enough, though I will continue to work on it further because I like a challenge. Knowing how bad it was in the past, and how tricky it can be to treat, I'm grateful that I can now live a 'normal' life free of the endless distress emetophobia causes.

Leaving school

Before we go into what life looks like now, let me catch you up on my story from where we left it. So, what happened when I finished school? Well, in the end, despite running on virtually no sleep or food, and powered by nothing other than adrenaline, out of control cortisol and a fair dose of bloody-mindedness, I got straight As in my exams and a place to read Geography at Cambridge University.

How I achieved that, I still don't know. The focus, anxiety, determination and self-punishment that went with the emetophobia seemed also to apply to my academic life and I forced myself to work ten or twelve hours a day every day of my last year of school. I couldn't stop. Couldn't allow myself the luxury of a break. It was another form of self-punishment and another symptom of perfectionism. Like I knew that I had to keep going endlessly because to stop and rest would mean to collapse completely.

The emetophobia probably did help with my studies in some twisted way but it came at a very heavy price. Not only did it destroy my health and wellbeing, but it also robbed me of a social life – in that sense it probably did aid my exam preparation. It robbed me of my teen years full stop. While having good grades is, of course, beneficial in life, health and wellbeing are so much more important.

Are my As and degree improving my life on a day-to-day basis now? No, of course not, though I did love my time at university. Do they help me when I'm trying to convince my six-year-old to eat his vegetables? Nope. Or when I'm vacuuming dog hair off the floor? No, not then either. Do they even offer any benefit when I'm writing a book? Not really. B grades and good health would have served me much better. In retrospect, looking after my wellbeing was far more important. But nothing could have convinced me of that at the time.

* * *

Inevitably, when my exams were over, I crumpled. I no longer had anything to keep me going. Everything I'd been working towards, focused on, and driven by, was over. I was so exhausted, drained, unwell and, well, broken, that once school finished, I went to bed and just cried for days and days. I couldn't sleep or read or get up – I just lay in bed and cried. I hadn't cried once all year – I'd been steely and emotionless – but the floodgates suddenly opened and then there was no stopping the tears.

Once the weeping had finally run its course, I just stared at the ceiling feeling nothing but grey bleakness. I'd given everything I had to give, and more, and now there was nothing left. There was just a sort of void where school and exams had been. What now?

Thankfully, I had a deferred place at university, so I had a year to get myself back on track before tackling university. I think I justified the year off to my soon-to-be tutor by persuading her that it was an important opportunity for seeing the wonders of the natural world and the marvels of planet Earth for myself before learning about them...

Yeah, that wasn't going to happen. I was too ill to leave the house, let alone go on a gap year to exotic and far-flung backpacking destinations. My gap year was for sorting my head out and nothing else.

Recovery

I can no longer remember how, or when, but around this point I stumbled on a condition called emetophobia online and everything started to fall into place. Until then I had believed I was suffering from some never-before-seen ailment of my own. I couldn't believe that I'd found a condition with a list of symptoms that exactly matched mine. I didn't realise it was possible for a mental health problem to fall into such a neat box. The list of symptoms I found even mentioned that people with emetophobia tend to carry mints with them. I always had Polos in my bag.

It was a huge relief to discover that I had a diagnosable illness. I was also, admittedly, slightly put out that I wasn't a special, one-of-a-kind mess.

Armed with this newfound knowledge, I had to sort myself out before my gap year was up. That summer I slept a lot, I sunbathed, I chilled with my friends in the garden, and I did a lot of reading. I finally allowed myself to rest, basically. There was no longer anything to drive myself towards, or for.

The rest and recovery time helped. Well, it was crucial. But, as I've said, the turning point finally came when the doctor agreed that, now I was an adult, I might benefit from anti-depressants and that the benefits should outweigh the risks of taking them. He put me on an SSRI and, once the initial side effects had worn off, things finally started to improve.

With the SSRI on board, I suddenly felt an interest in looking after myself properly and in trying to improve my wellbeing. I started doing some very gentle exercise – running round the block – and I started gradually to improve my diet. My food intake was still extremely restricted but without the pressure of having to go to school every day, and the fear of being sick at school, I started to eat a little more and a wider variety of foods. That helped. I started to gain a little bit of weight and must have been better nourished.

Inevitably, while my emetophobia wasn't specifically being treated, the rest, sleep, sunshine, food and removal of all pressure and work improved my wellbeing significantly – self-care, isn't it? I took a job at my best friend's parents' farm, and I enjoyed it. It was fun and that helped too. As did the opportunity for more chats and laughs with that bestie of mine.

University

Fifteen months after hitting rock bottom, finishing my exams and leaving school I went up to university, to start my Geography degree.

Inexplicably, I felt completely relaxed about leaving home and moving to this new city, new life and new experience. I've no idea why I wasn't nervous, but I wasn't. Maybe in a way I had nothing to lose – I'd been so unwell, and so unhappy, that things couldn't get any worse, so there was nothing to fear.

There was, also, another factor – during the summer before I went up to university, I acquired a psychiatrist in London who doubled my dose of SSRIs. He was employed to try to sort me out before university and his tactic seemed to be to drug me into oblivion. Any sign of ongoing anxiety, he threw drugs at. He also sent me to a therapist who started me on a course of CBT.

The psychiatrist started by doubling my medication dose and he would have gone further but I refused to take more. The impact of this was that I was very sleepy, but also very blasé and relaxed. Nothing fazed me any more – starting uni? Nope. Totally chilled about that. University exams? Nope, not those either. My primary concern with those was whether I could stay awake for the full three hours. Even the soul-destroying exam preparation? No. Not bothered. Just ate flapjacks and Haribo at my desk for a bit before succumbing to the temptation of my bed and another nap.

So, contrary to all expectations, I loved my time at university, gained more weight (thank you, flapjacks and Haribo), relaxed further, made masses of friends, partied, drank, sunbathed and gave as little energy to my studies as I could get away with. In other words, I was a 'normal' student living a 'normal' student life. And I was happy.

And now?

So where am I with all this now? Well, I like to consider myself cured of emetophobia but that isn't entirely accurate. I'm so used to it and have lived with it for so much of my life, that I find it tricky to tease out where it remains in my thought processes. It's the norm for me. I guess I'd have to spend a few days as a person who has never had emetophobia to be able to truly assess to what degree I still have it.

What I know is that it no longer causes me frequent distress.

I can now sit in cinemas and theatres without an iota of anxiety, I can eat in pubs and restaurants, I can sometimes eat at other people's houses, I can (and do) eat a varied, healthy, balanced diet and I have no anxiety about going out for the day, or about being somewhere with no bathroom.

The other huge ones are that I no longer feel nauseous or anxious in general and that I no longer plan my days around avoiding anxiety. I have also had two children and the mild morning sickness I experienced didn't faze me at all. I've had long spells off SSRIs altogether and muddled along okay without them. I've even survived the children having stomach bugs.

While it undoubtedly saved me, I still believe that SSRI medication is more of a sticking plaster than a magic bullet. Yes, it can be literally lifesaving in a crisis, and can make life liveable, but it doesn't address the underlying problems – only CBT and exposure therapy can do that. It didn't fix my emetophobia or erase the trauma that caused it, it just numbed me to it. Nor did it cure my anxiety or depression, it just masked them – like painkillers for a headache. A doctor friend explained to me once that it can allow you to relearn how to live without the phobia so that a phobia-free mindset becomes your norm. In that way, maybe it can aid genuine healing. Overall, though, I would view it more as a tool to make engaging with treatment easier and to make your life more manageable while you work on recovery.

So, now, fifteen years on, I'm still working on my emetophobia and perfectionism with a combination of lifestyle, CBT and, yes, a few SSRIs. You never know, maybe one day with enough hard work, determination and courage, I will be completely free of both the phobia and the medication. I'm gradually weaning down my SSRI dose again and I have finished my course of CBT. Only time will tell.

Coincidentally, while writing this chapter I've had a sickness bug and threw up for the first time in fifteen years. A friend pointed out to me that it was essentially research for the book.

What I learned was this: one might assume that for someone with emetophobia having a stomach bug would be the worst thing imaginable but, actually, it isn't. Not for me, anyway. The thing with emetophobia is that it's all about control and trying to reduce the risk of being sick. The anxiety comes from the possibility of being sick. So, for me at least, if I actually am sick I can kind of relax because the ship has already sailed. It's like I can finally give up the constant vigilance because it's too late.

I wish I could give you a clear roadmap for a smooth recovery journey. But it isn't that simple. How did I achieve my partial recovery? Well, I grew up and matured, I left school and exams and that context in which the phobia had developed, I made the most of the medication available, and I've had some brief spells of CBT and exposure therapy. I've also got hugely better at self-care and supporting my mental wellbeing through diet, exercise and lifestyle changes. I know that I will always have to be conscientious in the way I live my life to support my physical and mental health as best I can but, in truth, that probably applies to everyone.

Staying well

Now that you've gone through so much, and worked so hard to overcome your emetophobia, what can you do to stay well? What do the experts say about life after emetophobia, or emetophobia treatment?

To be in good health, both physically and mentally, everyone must make certain decisions about the way they live their life. We all know that if we eat well, exercise sensibly and get plenty of sleep we will be healthier than if we don't. It's no different for people who are recovering from emetophobia than for those with obesity, heart disease or type 2 diabetes. Indeed, it's no different for people with no significant health challenges. But what can you do specifically to keep your old emetophobia at bay?

Why not start by looking at the list of goals you made during CBT and see how you're getting on with them?[1] Can you now do things you weren't previously able to? If so, give yourself a huge pat on the back and take note of how much progress you've made – it's easy to forget how things used to be and, therefore, not to notice how much better you are. Don't fixate on the challenges you still have – take a moment to recognise and appreciate your progress. Then, if you're doing well with your original targets, maybe set yourself some new and more ambitious ones – that's the way to make further progress. Or, if there are some that have fallen by the wayside, try challenging yourself again.

Staying healthy is a lifelong journey which requires you to continue challenging yourself frequently to keep your emetophobia at bay[2] – sadly, you probably can't expect to do a few months of therapy and then be able to skip off into the sunset cured for life. Keep up those challenges and, with a bit of luck, you will keep getting better and better.

However hard you work, recovery doesn't tend to be a linear process, and setbacks are par for the course. Don't despair if you meet one. It's normal and natural that it's happened. The key is how you respond to it. Don't let it knock you off course. If you recognise that it's happened, and why, you will soon get back on track. If you're still struggling after a week or two, maybe you could organise an extra session with your therapist to go through it, or chat to a friend who is understanding. Setting yourself some new exposure challenges can also help.[3] Often, though, a good night's sleep and a new day is all it takes.

The main thing to remember is that the best way to maintain the gains you've made is to keep putting them into practice.[4]

For example, if you've got to the point where you can eat in restaurants, don't achieve it and then leave it a year before doing it again – make sure you go as often as possible. Or if you've cracked going on public transport, ditch the car and use buses and trains as often as possible. That way, you won't slip back into old, emetophobic habits and lose the gains you've worked so hard for.

As part of continuing to challenge yourself, it's crucial to explain to those around you that, however well meaning it is, they mustn't shield you from things that make you anxious.[5] For example, they mustn't lie to you about whether they feel unwell. To get better, and to stay better, being exposed to this sort of information and uncertainty is crucial. Therapists recommend that you continue to practise exposures until at least six months after you technically finish treatment.[6]

To help you stay on the path to recovery, you could appoint someone to support you – a parent or partner would be an obvious choice. This person may well be the same person who supported you through treatment. With a bit of guidance and training, having someone in this role can be extremely helpful. They need to be kind and patient as well as consistent. They mustn't get angry or frustrated as this makes things worse. They are more like a guide who can help steer you back to the path of recovery if you have a wobble. This isn't an easy role for someone to fill as they mustn't offer any reassurance or comfort – this could enable the continuation of the phobia and prevent you learning to manage your anxiety on your own. They must allow you to solve your own problems and must proceed as though you have no anxiety, regardless of what you ask them to do. For example, if you ask them to overcook the dinner, they should refuse and should cook it correctly.[7]

Ellie said, 'Even though I no longer have emetophobia, I still use the techniques I learned in CBT. I use a lot of breathing exercises to calm myself down. If I start to feel a bit panicky, I turn to what I was taught.'

She added, 'Sometimes I take five minutes out to get some fresh air and have a drink of water. Those are the things I still use that mean it's basically treated now.'

My top tips for staying well after emetophobia

- Look after all aspects of your health by eating well, exercising, getting plenty of sleep and spending time with friends and family.
- When you've cracked a new skill – such as going on boats – don't assume you've now done that and can forget it. Keep practising your new skill so you don't lose it again.
- Keep challenging yourself and keep making the challenges slightly more difficult and more ambitious.
- Surround yourself with people who are understanding and respectful of your anxieties but who don't pander to them – you're best off with people who challenge you with love and kindness. People who shelter you

from things they think will make you anxious are probably trying to be kind, or to avoid unnecessary stress, but aren't doing you any favours in the long run.

- Work hard on your relationships to ensure you are surrounded by supportive people who will celebrate your victories with you, support you through difficult times and always be there if you need to talk.
- Celebrate little wins and keep looking for more!

The conclusion

So, there you have it. We've explored what emetophobia is, who has it, where it comes from, how it impacts people's lives, how to recover and how to stay better.

Emetophobia is a very difficult condition to live with and can have a devastating impact on people's lives. It isn't easy or quick to treat but it is treatable, and, with a bit of work and dedication, you can get better. So, seize the day, find a therapist – or, if that isn't possible, a CBT self-help book and a good mate – who can help you tackle those exposures with courage. You will reap the rewards.

Don't allow yourself to be knocked by bad days or setbacks. Just keep plugging on and challenging yourself – the rewards will be enormous, and you can and will transform your life.

Never forget that you aren't walking this road alone – emetophobia is surprisingly common – thousands of people have tackled it before you, are tackling it now, and will tackle it in the future. All these people, including me, understand what you are going through, and how hard it is, and are rooting for you.

I've been thinking of you as I've been writing this book and will continue to think of you as it's released into the world. I wish it could have contained a simple secret to escaping emetophobia overnight but, sadly, that isn't how life, or this condition, works.

I've tried to be completely open and honest about my own experience and have presented a bitesize rattle through the information currently available on emetophobia. It's a topic that has been gaining much more attention and interest in recent years so the amount and quality of information available is increasing all the time. I hope this will also lead to further research into the phobia and how best to treat it. So, watch this space and let's both hope for an easier solution to be discovered soon.

For now, good luck – you can do it!

References

Introduction

1 Russ, D. & Christie, A. (2023) *Emetophobia: Understanding and Treating Fear of Vomiting in Children and Adults*. London: Jessica Kingsley Publishers, p.91.

Chapter 1

1 Anxiety UK (2024) *Emetophobia*. Accessed on 18/08/2024 at www.anxietyuk.org.uk/anxiety-type/emetophobia

2 Keyes, A. & Veale, D. (2022) *Free Yourself from Emetophobia*. London: Jessica Kingsley Publishers, p.21.

3 Russ, D. & Christie, A. (2023) *Emetophobia: Understanding and Treating Fear of Vomiting in Children and Adults*. London: Jessica Kingsley Publishers.

4 Russ, D. & Christie, A. (2023) *Emetophobia: Understanding and Treating Fear of Vomiting in Children and Adults*. London: Jessica Kingsley Publishers.

5 Russ, D. & Christie, A. (2023) *Emetophobia: Understanding and Treating Fear of Vomiting in Children and Adults*. London: Jessica Kingsley Publishers.

6 Keyes, A. & Veale, D. (2022) *Free Yourself from Emetophobia*. London: Jessica Kingsley Publishers, p.45.

7 Russ, D. & Christie, A. (2023) *Emetophobia: Understanding and Treating Fear of Vomiting in Children and Adults*. London: Jessica Kingsley Publishers.

8 Goodman, K. (2020) *The Emetophobia Manual: Free Yourself from the Fear of Vomit and Reclaim Your Life*. California: Anxiety and OCD Treatment of the Valley.

9 Russ, D. & Christie, A. (2023) *Emetophobia: Understanding and Treating Fear of Vomiting in Children and Adults*. London: Jessica Kingsley Publishers.

10 NHS (2023) Panic Disorder. Accessed on 30/09/2025 at www.nhs.uk/mental-health/conditions/panic-disorder
11 Keyes, A. & Veale, D. (2022) *Free Yourself from Emetophobia*. London: Jessica Kingsley Publishers.
12 Keyes, A. & Veale, D. (2022) *Free Yourself from Emetophobia*. London: Jessica Kingsley Publishers.
13 EmetAction (2023) What Is Emetophobia? Accessed on 21/04/2025 at https://emetaction.org/what-is-emetophobia
14 EmetAction (2023) What Is Emetophobia? Accessed on 21/04/2025 at https://emetaction.org/what-is-emetophobia
15 NHS (2022) Overview – Phobias. Accessed on 25/04/2025 at www.nhs.uk/mental-health/conditions/phobias/overview
16 Keyes, A. & Veale, D. (2022) *Free Yourself from Emetophobia*. London: Jessica Kingsley Publishers.
17 Keyes, A. & Veale, D. (2022) *Free Yourself from Emetophobia*. London: Jessica Kingsley Publishers.
18 Keyes, A. & Veale, D. (2022) *Free Yourself from Emetophobia*. London: Jessica Kingsley Publishers.
19 Russ, D. & Christie, A. (2023) *Emetophobia: Understanding and Treating Fear of Vomiting in Children and Adults*. London: Jessica Kingsley Publishers.
20 Keyes, A. & Veale, D. (2022) *Free Yourself from Emetophobia*. London: Jessica Kingsley Publishers.
21 Keyes, A. & Veale, D. (2022) *Free Yourself from Emetophobia*. London: Jessica Kingsley Publishers.
22 Russ, D. & Christie, A. (2023) *Emetophobia: Understanding and Treating Fear of Vomiting in Children and Adults*. London: Jessica Kingsley Publishers.
23 Keyes, A. & Veale, D. (2022) *Free Yourself from Emetophobia*. London: Jessica Kingsley Publishers.
24 Keyes, A. & Veale, D. (2022) *Free Yourself from Emetophobia*. London: Jessica Kingsley Publishers.
25 Russ, D. & Christie, A. (2023) *Emetophobia: Understanding and Treating Fear of Vomiting in Children and Adults*. London: Jessica Kingsley Publishers.
26 Keyes, A. & Veale, D. (2022) *Free Yourself from Emetophobia*. London: Jessica Kingsley Publishers.
27 Keyes, A. & Veale, D. (2022) *Free Yourself from Emetophobia*. London: Jessica Kingsley Publishers.
28 Russ, D. & Christie, A. (2023) *Emetophobia: Understanding and Treating Fear of Vomiting in Children and Adults*. London: Jessica Kingsley Publishers.
29 Keyes, A. & Veale, D. (2022) *Free Yourself from Emetophobia*. London: Jessica Kingsley Publishers.

30 Keyes, A. & Veale, D. (2022) *Free Yourself from Emetophobia*. London: Jessica Kingsley Publishers.

Chapter 2

1 Keyes, A. & Veale, D. (2022) *Free Yourself from Emetophobia*. London: Jessica Kingsley Publishers.
2 Chatterjee, R. (2018) *The 4 Pillar Plan: How to Relax, Eat, Move, Sleep Your Way to a Longer, Healthier Life*. London: Penguin Random House UK, p.90.
3 Chatterjee, R. (2018) *The 4 Pillar Plan: How to Relax, Eat, Move, Sleep Your Way to a Longer, Healthier Life*. London: Penguin Random House UK, p.50.
4 Chatterjee, R. (2023) #336 *How Trauma Impacts Your Physical Health & How to Heal from it with Dr Bessel van der Kolk* [Feel Better, Live More] 15 February 2023.
5 Chatterjee, R. (2023) #336 *How Trauma Impacts Your Physical Health & How to Heal from it with Dr Bessel van der Kolk* [Feel Better, Live More] 15 February 2023.

Chapter 3

1 Keyes, A. & Veale, D. (2022) *Free Yourself from Emetophobia*. London: Jessica Kingsley Publishers.
2 Russ, D. & Christie, A. (2023) *Emetophobia: Understanding and Treating Fear of Vomiting in Children and Adults*. London: Jessica Kingsley Publishers.
3 Russ, D. & Christie, A. (2023) *Emetophobia: Understanding and Treating Fear of Vomiting in Children and Adults*. London: Jessica Kingsley Publishers, p.52.
4 Russ, D. & Christie, A. (2023) *Emetophobia: Understanding and Treating Fear of Vomiting in Children and Adults*. London: Jessica Kingsley Publishers.
5 Keyes, A. & Veale, D. (2022) *Free Yourself from Emetophobia*. London: Jessica Kingsley Publishers.
6 Russ, D. & Christie, A. (2023) *Emetophobia: Understanding and Treating Fear of Vomiting in Children and Adults*. London: Jessica Kingsley Publishers.
7 Goodman, K. (2020) *The Emetophobia Manual: Free Yourself from the Fear of Vomit and Reclaim Your Life*. California: Anxiety and OCD Treatment of the Valley.
8 NHS (2023) Calculate Your Body Mass Index (BMI) for Adults. Accessed on 21/04/2025 at www.nhs.uk/health-assessment-tools/calculate-your-body-mass-index/calculate-bmi-for-adults
9 NHS (2023) Symptoms: Malnutrition. Accessed on 21/04/2025 at www.nhs.uk/conditions/malnutrition/symptoms

10 Nall, R. (2023) What are the risks of being underweight? London: Medical News Today. Accessed on 21/04/2025 at www.medicalnewstoday.com/articles/321612
11 Keyes, A. & Veale, D. (2022) *Free Yourself from Emetophobia*. London: Jessica Kingsley Publishers.
12 Psychology Today (2023) How to Break the Malnutrition and Mental Function Deadlock. Accessed on 17/06/2025 at www.psychologytoday.com/us/blog/a-hunger-artist/202306/how-to-break-the-malnutrition-and-mental-function-deadlock
13 Keyes, A. & Veale, D. (2022) *Free Yourself from Emetophobia*. London: Jessica Kingsley Publishers.

Chapter 4

1 Goodman, K. (2020) *The Emetophobia Manual: Free Yourself from the Fear of Vomit and Reclaim Your Life*. California: Anxiety and OCD Treatment of the Valley.
2 Keyes, A. & Veale, D. (2022) *Free Yourself from Emetophobia*. London: Jessica Kingsley Publishers.
3 Goodman, K. (2020) *The Emetophobia Manual: Free Yourself from the Fear of Vomit and Reclaim Your Life*. California: Anxiety and OCD Treatment of the Valley.
4 Russ, D. & Christie, A. (2023) *Emetophobia: Understanding and Treating Fear of Vomiting in Children and Adults*. London: Jessica Kingsley Publishers.
5 Chatterjee, R. (2018) *The Stress Solution*. London: Penguin Random House UK.

Chapter 5

1 Chatterjee, R. (2018) *The 4 Pillar Plan: How to Relax, Eat, Move, Sleep Your Way to a Longer, Healthier Life*. London: Penguin Random House UK.
2 Chatterjee, R. (2018) *The Stress Solution*. London: Penguin Random House UK.
3 Mind (2023) Disability Discrimination. Accessed on 08/05/2025 at www.mind.org.uk/information-support/legal-rights/disability-discrimination/complaining-about-disability-discrimination
4 Mind (2023) Disability Discrimination. Accessed on 08/05/2025 at www.mind.org.uk/information-support/legal-rights/disability-discrimination/complaining-about-disability-discrimination
5 Mind (2023) Disability Discrimination. Accessed on 08/05/2025 at www.mind.org.uk/information-support/legal-rights/disability-discrimination/complaining-about-disability-discrimination

6 Mind (2023) Disability Discrimination. Accessed on 08/05/2025 at www.mind.org.uk/information-support/legal-rights/disability-discrimination/complaining-about-disability-discrimination
7 Mind (2023) Disability Discrimination. Accessed on 08/05/2025 at www.mind.org.uk/information-support/legal-rights/disability-discrimination/complaining-about-disability-discrimination
8 Keyes, A. & Veale, D. (2022) *Free Yourself from Emetophobia*. London: Jessica Kingsley Publishers, p.27.

Chapter 6

1 Chatterjee, R. (2018) *The Stress Solution*. London: Penguin Random House UK.
2 Chatterjee, R. (2018) *The Stress Solution*. London: Penguin Random House UK.
3 Chatterjee, R. (2018) *The Stress Solution*. London: Penguin Random House UK.
4 Lawrie, E. (2025) Can AI therapists really be an alternative to human help? BBC InDepth. Accessed on 04/08/2025 at www.bbc.co.uk/news/articles/ced2ywg7246o
5 Spytska, L. (2025) The use of artificial intelligence in psychotherapy: Development of intelligent therapeutic systems. *BMC Psychology*, 13, 175.
6 Lawrie, E. (2025) Can AI therapists really be an alternative to human help? BBC InDepth. Accessed on 04/08/2025 at www.bbc.co.uk/news/articles/ced2ywg7246o
7 Taylor, J. (2025) AI chatbots are becoming popular alternatives to therapy. But they may worsen mental health crises, experts warn. *The Guardian*. Accessed on 04/08/2025 at www.theguardian.com/australia-news/2025/aug/03/ai-chatbot-as-therapy-alternative-mental-health-crises-ntwnfb
8 Abby (2025) *AI Therapy in Your Pocket*. Accessed on 12/08/2025 at https://abby.gg

Chapter 7

1 Russ, D. & Christie, A. (2023) *Emetophobia: Understanding and Treating Fear of Vomiting in Children and Adults*. London: Jessica Kingsley Publishers, p.105.
2 Keyes, A. & Veale, D. (2022) *Free Yourself from Emetophobia*. London: Jessica Kingsley Publishers.
3 Russ, D. & Christie, A. (2023) *Emetophobia: Understanding and Treating Fear of Vomiting in Children and Adults*. London: Jessica Kingsley Publishers, p.105.
4 British Association for Behavioural and Cognitive Psychotherapies (n.d.) Looking for a CBT Therapist? Accessed on 12/01/2026 at https://babcp.com/what-is-cbt/mental-health-support-services-information

5 British Association for Counselling and Psychotherapy (BACP) (n.d.) Accessed on 12/01/2026 at www.bacp.co.uk

6 United Kingdom Council for Psychotherapy (UKCP) (n.d.) Find a Therapist. Accessed on 12/01/2026 at www.psychotherapy.org.uk

7 Emetophobia Help (2025) How to Find a Therapist. Accessed on 08/11/2025 at https://emetophobiahelp.org/how-to-find-a-therapist

8 Psychology Today (n.d.) Accessed on 12/01/2026 at www.psychologytoday.com/gb

9 Russ, D. & Christie, A. (2023) *Emetophobia: Understanding and Treating Fear of Vomiting in Children and Adults*. London: Jessica Kingsley Publishers, p.25.

10 Russ, D. & Christie, A. (2023) *Emetophobia: Understanding and Treating Fear of Vomiting in Children and Adults*. London: Jessica Kingsley Publishers, p.105.

11 Keyes, A. & Veale, D. (2022) *Free Yourself from Emetophobia*. London: Jessica Kingsley Publishers.

12 Russ, D. & Christie, A. (2023) *Emetophobia: Understanding and Treating Fear of Vomiting in Children and Adults*. London: Jessica Kingsley Publishers.

13 Keyes, A. & Veale, D. (2022) *Free Yourself from Emetophobia*. London: Jessica Kingsley Publishers.

14 Russ, D. & Christie, A. (2023) *Emetophobia: Understanding and Treating Fear of Vomiting in Children and Adults*. London: Jessica Kingsley Publishers.

15 Goodman, K. (2020) *The Emetophobia Manual: Free Yourself from the Fear of Vomit and Reclaim Your Life*. California: Anxiety and OCD Treatment of the Valley.

16 Russ, D. & Christie, A. (2023) *Emetophobia: Understanding and Treating Fear of Vomiting in Children and Adults*. London: Jessica Kingsley Publishers.

17 Russ, D. & Christie, A. (2023) *Emetophobia: Understanding and Treating Fear of Vomiting in Children and Adults*. London: Jessica Kingsley Publishers.

18 Russ, D. & Christie, A. (2023) *Emetophobia: Understanding and Treating Fear of Vomiting in Children and Adults*. London: Jessica Kingsley Publishers.

19 Keyes, A. & Veale, D. (2022) *Free Yourself from Emetophobia*. London: Jessica Kingsley Publishers.

20 Russ, D. & Christie, A. (2023) *Emetophobia: Understanding and Treating Fear of Vomiting in Children and Adults*. London: Jessica Kingsley Publishers.

21 Keyes, A. & Veale, D. (2022) *Free Yourself from Emetophobia*. London: Jessica Kingsley Publishers, p.8.

22 Keyes, A. & Veale, D. (2022) *Free Yourself from Emetophobia*. London: Jessica Kingsley Publishers.
23 Keyes, A. & Veale, D. (2022) *Free Yourself from Emetophobia*. London: Jessica Kingsley Publishers.
24 Russ, D. & Christie, A. (2023) *Emetophobia: Understanding and Treating Fear of Vomiting in Children and Adults*. London: Jessica Kingsley Publishers.
25 Keyes, A. & Veale, D. (2022) *Free Yourself from Emetophobia*. London: Jessica Kingsley Publishers.
26 Russ, D. & Christie, A. (2023) *Emetophobia: Understanding and Treating Fear of Vomiting in Children and Adults*. London: Jessica Kingsley Publishers.
27 Keyes, A. & Veale, D. (2022) *Free Yourself from Emetophobia*. London: Jessica Kingsley Publishers.
28 Keyes, A. & Veale, D. (2022) *Free Yourself from Emetophobia*. London: Jessica Kingsley Publishers.
29 Keyes, A. & Veale, D. (2022) *Free Yourself from Emetophobia*. London: Jessica Kingsley Publishers.
30 Keyes, A. & Veale, D. (2022) *Free Yourself from Emetophobia*. London: Jessica Kingsley Publishers.
31 Keyes, A. & Veale, D. (2022) *Free Yourself from Emetophobia*. London: Jessica Kingsley Publishers.
32 Keyes, A. & Veale, D. (2022) *Free Yourself from Emetophobia*. London: Jessica Kingsley Publishers.
33 Keyes, A. & Veale, D. (2022) *Free Yourself from Emetophobia*. London: Jessica Kingsley Publishers.
34 Keyes, A. & Veale, D. (2022) *Free Yourself from Emetophobia*. London: Jessica Kingsley Publishers.
35 Russ, D. & Christie, A. (2023) *Emetophobia: Understanding and Treating Fear of Vomiting in Children and Adults*. London: Jessica Kingsley Publishers.
36 Russ, D. & Christie, A. (2023) *Emetophobia: Understanding and Treating Fear of Vomiting in Children and Adults*. London: Jessica Kingsley Publishers.

Chapter 8

1 Chatterjee, R. (2018) *The 4 Pillar Plan: How to Relax, Eat, Move, Sleep Your Way to a Longer, Healthier Life*. London: Penguin Random House UK, p.8.
2 Chatterjee, R. (2018) *The 4 Pillar Plan: How to Relax, Eat, Move, Sleep Your Way to a Longer, Healthier Life*. London: Penguin Random House UK, p.10.
3 Chatterjee, R. (2018) *The Stress Solution*. London: Penguin Random House UK.

4 Chatterjee, R. (2018) *The 4 Pillar Plan: How to Relax, Eat, Move, Sleep Your Way to a Longer, Healthier Life*. London: Penguin Random House UK.
5 Chatterjee, R. (2018) *The 4 Pillar Plan: How to Relax, Eat, Move, Sleep Your Way to a Longer, Healthier Life*. London: Penguin Random House UK.
6 Walker, M. (2017) *Why We Sleep*. New York, NY: Schriber.
7 Chatterjee, R. (2018) *The 4 Pillar Plan: How to Relax, Eat, Move, Sleep Your Way to a Longer, Healthier Life*. London: Penguin Random House UK.
8 Chatterjee, R. (2018) *The 4 Pillar Plan: How to Relax, Eat, Move, Sleep Your Way to a Longer, Healthier Life*. London: Penguin Random House UK.
9 Chatterjee, R. (2018) *The 4 Pillar Plan: How to Relax, Eat, Move, Sleep Your Way to a Longer, Healthier Life*. London: Penguin Random House UK.
10 Chatterjee, R. (2018) *The Stress Solution*. London: Penguin Random House UK.
11 Chatterjee, R. (2018) *The Stress Solution*. London: Penguin Random House UK.
12 Chatterjee, R. (2018) *The Stress Solution*. London: Penguin Random House UK.
13 Chatterjee, R. (2018) *The Stress Solution*. London: Penguin Random House UK.

Chapter 9

1 Keyes, A. & Veale, D. (2022) *Free Yourself from Emetophobia*. London: Jessica Kingsley Publishers.
2 Keyes, A. & Veale, D. (2022) *Free Yourself from Emetophobia*. London: Jessica Kingsley Publishers.
3 Keyes, A. & Veale, D. (2022) *Free Yourself from Emetophobia*. London: Jessica Kingsley Publishers.
4 Keyes, A. & Veale, D. (2022) *Free Yourself from Emetophobia*. London: Jessica Kingsley Publishers.
5 Russ, D. & Christie, A. (2023) *Emetophobia: Understanding and Treating Fear of Vomiting in Children and Adults*. London: Jessica Kingsley Publishers.
6 Russ, D. & Christie, A. (2023) *Emetophobia: Understanding and Treating Fear of Vomiting in Children and Adults*. London: Jessica Kingsley Publishers.
7 Russ, D. & Christie, A. (2023) *Emetophobia: Understanding and Treating Fear of Vomiting in Children and Adults*. London: Jessica Kingsley Publishers.

Bibliography

Abby (2025) *AI Therapy in Your Pocket*. Accessed on 12/08/2025 at https://abby.gg

Anxiety UK (2024) *Emetophobia*. Accessed on 18/08/2024 at www.anxietyuk.org.uk/anxiety-type/emetophobia

British Association for Behavioural and Cognitive Psychotherapies (n.d.) Looking for a CBT Therapist? Accessed on 12/01/2026 at https://babcp.com

British Association for Counselling and Psychotherapy (BACP) (n.d.) Accessed on 12/01/2026 at www.bacp.co.uk

Bryon, T. (2025, April 7) 'Ask Professor Tanya Byron: My daughter has developed a vomit phobia that is ruining her life.' Times2, *The Times*.

Chatterjee, R. (2018) *The Stress Solution*. London: Penguin Random House UK.

Chatterjee, R. (2023) #336 *How Trauma Impacts Your Physical Health & How to Heal from it with Dr Bessel van der Kolk* [Feel Better, Live More] 15 February 2023.

Chatterjee, R. (2025) #563 *Rethinking Mental Health: What the Science Actually Says about Depression, the Side Effects of Antidepressants & Finding Balance with Professor Joanna Moncrieff* [Feel Better, Life More] 10 June 2025.

EmetAction (2023) *What Is Emetophobia?* Accessed 21/04/2025 at https://emetaction.org/what-is-emetophobia

Emetophobia Help (2025) *How To Find A Therapist*. Accessed on 08/11/2025 at https://emetophobiahelp.org/how-to-find-a-therapist/

Keyes, A. & Veale, D. (2022) *Free Yourself from Emetophobia*. London: Jessica Kingsley Publishers.

Goodman, K. (2020) *The Emetophobia Manual: Free Yourself from the Fear of Vomit and Reclaim Your Life*. California: Anxiety and OCD Treatment of the Valley.

Lawrie, E. (2025) Can AI therapists really be an alternative to human help? BBC InDepth. Accessed on 04/08/2025 at www.bbc.co.uk/news/articles/ced2ywg7246o

Mafi, A. (2025) The risks and benefits of AI therapy tools. *BMJ*, 389, r821. Accessed on 04/08/2025 at www.bmj.com/content/389/bmj.r821

Mind (2017) Mental Health Problems – An Introduction. Accessed on 05/05/2025 at www.mind.org.uk/information-support/types-of-mental-health-problems/mental-health-problems-introduction/stigma-misconceptions

Mind (2023) Disability Discrimination. Accessed on 08/05/2025 at www.mind.org.uk/information-support/legal-rights/disability-discrimination/complaining-about-disability-discrimination

Nall, R. (2023) What are the risks of being underweight? London: Medical News Today. Accessed on 21/04/2025 at www.medicalnewstoday.com/articles/321612

NHS (2022a) About Citalopram. Accessed on 18/08/2024 at www.nhs.uk/medicines/citalopram/about-citalopram

NHS (2022b) Overview – Phobias. Accessed on 25/04/2025 at www.nhs.uk/mental-health/conditions/phobias/overview

NHS (2022c) Side Effects of Citalopram. Accessed on 18/08/2024 at www.nhs.uk/medicines/citalopram/side-effects-of-citalopram

NHS (2023a) Calculate Your Body Mass Index (BMI) for Adults. Accessed on 21/04/2025 at www.nhs.uk/health-assessment-tools/calculate-your-body-mass-index/calculate-bmi-for-adults

NHS (2023b) Healthy Ways to Gain Weight. Accessed on 21/04/2025 at www.nhs.uk/live-well/healthy-weight/managing-your-weight/healthy-ways-to-gain-weight

NHS (2023c) Panic Disorder. Accessed on 30/09/2025 at www.nhs.uk/mental-health/conditions/panic-disorder

NHS (2023d) Self-Assessment Tool. Accessed on 19/05/2023 at https://checkwellbeing.leadershipacademy.nhs.uk/check-my-wellbeing/psychological-wellbeing-checker/#gf_21

NHS (2023e) Symptoms: Malnutrition. Accessed on 21/04/2025 at www.nhs.uk/conditions/malnutrition/symptoms

NHS (2024) Overview – Anorexia nervosa. Accessed on 18/08/2024 at www.nhs.uk/mental-health/conditions/anorexia/overview

Psychology Today (2023) How to Break the Malnutrition and Mental Function Deadlock. Accessed on 17/06/2025 at www.psychologytoday.com/us/blog/a-hunger-artist/202306/how-to-break-the-malnutrition-and-mental-function-deadlock

Russ, R. & Christie, A. (2023) *Emetophobia: Understanding and Treating Fear of Vomiting in Children and Adults*. London: Jessica Kingsley Publishers.

Spytska, L. (2025) The use of artificial intelligence in psychotherapy: Development of intelligent therapeutic systems. *BMC Psychology*, 13, 175.

Taylor, J. (2025) AI chatbots are becoming popular alternatives to therapy. But they may worsen mental health crises, experts warn. *The Guardian*.

Accessed on 04/08/2025 at www.theguardian.com/australia-news/2025/aug/03/ai-chatbot-as-therapy-alternative-mental-health-crises-ntwnfb

United Kingdom Council for Psychotherapy (UKCP) (n.d.) Find a Therapist. Accessed on 12/01/2026 at www.psychotherapy.org.uk

Walker, M. (2017) *Why We Sleep*. New York, NY: Schriber.

Further Reading

Books

- *Free Yourself from Emetophobia: A CBT Self-Help Guide for a Fear of Vomiting* by Dr Alexandra Keyes and Professor David Veale. London: Jessica Kingsley Publishers, 2022.
- *Living with Emetophobia: Coping with Extreme Fear of Vomiting* by Nicolette Heaton-Harris. London: Jessica Kingsley Publishers, 2007.
- *The Emetophobia Manual: Free Yourself from the Fear of Vomit and Reclaim Your Life* by Ken Goodman. California: Anxiety and OCD Treatment of the Valley, 2020.
- *Emetophobia: Understanding and Treating Fear of Vomiting in Children and Adults* by Dr David Russ and Anna Christie. London: Jessica Kingsley Publishers, 2023.
- *The 4 Pillar Plan: How to Relax, Eat, Move, Sleep Your Way to a Longer, Healthier Life* by Dr Rangan Chatterjee. London: Penguin Random House UK, 2018.
- *The Stress Solution* by Dr Rangan Chatterjee. London: Penguin Random House UK, 2018.

Workbooks

- *Emetophobia Workbook: CBT and ERP Worksheets to Break the Fear of Vomiting* by Dario Jeyco, 2023.
- *Emetophobia: An ERP Activity Book* by Dr Erin Neely, 2022.
- *Scared to Be Sick: A Self-Help Workbook for Emetophobia* by Samantha Watkins, Independent Publishing Network, 2018.

Websites

- EmetAction – www.emetaction.org
- British Association for Counselling and Psychotherapy – www.bacp.co.uk
- The UK Council for Psychotherapy – www.psychotherapy.org.uk
- Anxiety UK – www.anxietyuk.org.uk
- YoungMinds – www.youngminds.org.uk
- OCD-UK – www.ocduk.org
- Anxiety & Depression Association of America – https://adaa.org
- Emetophobia Help – https://emetophobiahelp.org
- Emetophobia Resources – Anna Christie and Dr. David Russ – https://emetophobia.net
- Psychology Today – www.psychologytoday.com